MILD
COGNITIVE
IMPAIRMENT

MILD
COGNITIVE
IMPAIRMENT

Aging to Alzheimer's Disease

Edited by
RONALD C. PETERSEN, Ph.D., M.D.

Cora Kanow Professor of Alzheimer's Disease Research
Mayo Medical School
Alzheimer's Disease Research Center
Mayo Clinic and Mayo Foundation
Rochester, Minnesota

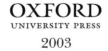

OXFORD
UNIVERSITY PRESS
2003

OXFORD

UNIVERSITY PRESS

Oxford   New York
Auckland   Bangkok   Buenos Aires   Cape Town   Chennai
Dar es Salaam   Delhi   Hong Kong   Istanbul   Karachi   Kolkata
Kuala Lumpur   Madrid   Melbourne   Mexico City   Mumbai
Nairobi   São Paulo   Shanghai   Taipei   Tokyo   Toronto

Published by Oxford University Press, Inc.
198 Madison Avenue, New York, New York 10016
http://www.oup-usa.org

Oxford is a registered trademark of Oxford University Press

Library of Congress Cataloging-in-Publication Data
Mild cognitive impairment : aging to Alzheimer's disease /
edited by Ronald C. Petersen.
p. ; cm.   Includes bibliographical references and index.
ISBN 0-19-512342-5
1. Cognition disorders in old age.   2. Alzheimer's disease.   3. Aging.
I. Petersen, Ronald C., 1946–
[DNLM: 1. Cognition Disorders—diagnosis—Aged.   2. Aging—psychology.
3. Alzheimer Disease—prevention & control.
WT 150 M641 2003]
RC553.C64 M54 2003
618.97'68—dc21   2002070435

2 4 6 8 9 7 5 3 1

Printed in the United States of America
on acid-free paper

To Diane, Lindsay, and Matthew

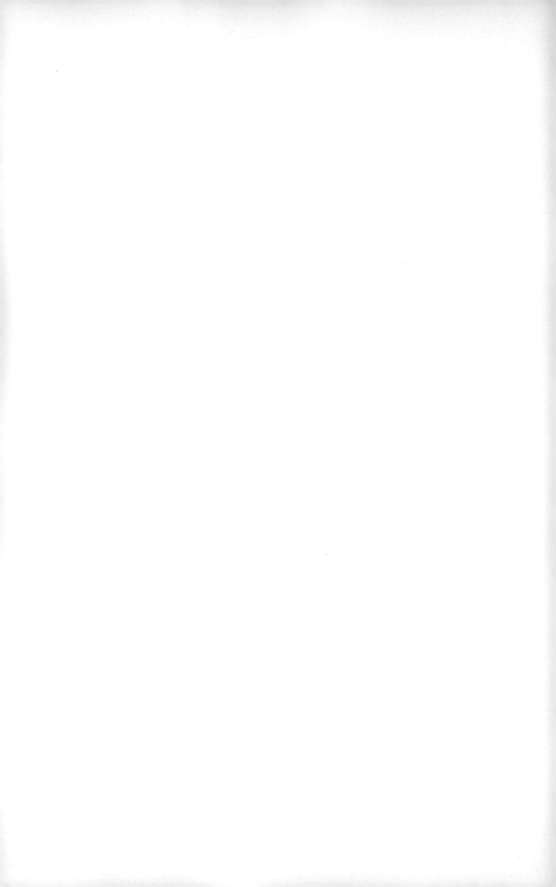

PREFACE

Research on aging and dementia is evolving toward an improved understanding of cognitive dysfunction at its earliest stage. This topic is becoming increasingly important as baby-boomers advance into the age at which they are at risk for Alzheimer's disease. Clinical investigators have been focusing on the borderland between cognitive changes of normal aging and very early Alzheimer's disease for several years, but the precise characterization of this intermediate condition has been challenging.

Mild cognitive impairment is a term used to describe this transitional zone between aging and very early AD. Presumably Alzheimer's disease develops over many years, perhaps decades, and it is likely that there is a gradual phase through which those individuals destined to develop Alzheimer's disease will progress. Mild cognitive impairment has been studied for many years, and a great deal is known about the clinical characterization, outcome, and predictors of progression. However, as the concept is investigated more intensively, problems surface. There is likely to be both clinical and etiological heterogeneity. The clinical criteria for mild cognitive impairment and the nature of its underlying neuropathology are controversial.

Nevertheless, there is also agreement among many clinicians and researchers that mild cognitive impairment is a useful concept which is moving the field forward. As research on aging and dementia moves toward prevention, the concept of mild cognitive impairment becomes useful in characterizing persons at their earliest stage of clinical impairment. While disease-modifying treatments are currently not available, many are being investigated, and it is vitally important to have well-characterized clinical populations available to allow assessment of these agents. In many respects, a cohort of mild cognitive impairment subjects is ideal for the evaluation of disease modifying treatments, since these subjects are minimally impaired and therefore quite able to cooperate with testing. In addition, their rate of clinical progression is well known. There are presently several clinical trials underway for the treatment of mild cognitive impairment, so the concept is receiving a great deal of attention worldwide.

The contributors to this volume were asked to address their topics from the perspective of the transitional zone between normal aging and very early cognitive impairment. The chapters deal with clinical criteria, cognitive characterization, non-cognitive symptoms, neuropsychological testing, structural and functional neuroimaging, neuropathology, biomarkers, and treatments. The initial chapter outlines the conceptual nature of the field of mild cognitive impairment as it currently exists and attempts to address some of the controversial areas. The clinical chapters provide a historical perspective and review existing studies. The neuropsychology chapters address two approaches to the cognitive characterization of normal subjects, an important concept that provides the background against which the boundaries of mild cognitive impairment can be defined. Since neuroimaging has become essential in the evaluation of subjects in the field of aging and dementia, two chapters deal with structural and functional aspects of the neuroimaging of individuals with mild cognitive impairment. The neuropathology of mild cognitive impairment is very important since it relates to the controversial question of whether subjects with these clinical features already have the neuropathological substrate of Alzheimer's disease or whether they represent a transitional condition with only incipient neuropathological features of Alzheimer's disease. Biomarkers are discussed as important adjuncts in making the clinical diagnosis of mild cognitive impairment and their present status is summarized. Finally, the treatments for mild cognitive impairment are evolving, and the final chapter reviews the current status of Alzheimer's disease therapy and outlines trials that are underway for mild cognitive impairment. Each of these contributions highlights the known data and remaining challenge with respect to this transitional condition. While there is no consensus on the concept of mild cognitive impairment at present, this volume is intended to outline the salient topics and discuss relevant issues from multiple perspectives.

Rochester, Minnesota   R.C.P.

CONTENTS

CONTRIBUTORS

MARILYN S. ALBERT, PH.D.
Professor of Psychiatry and
  Neurology
Harvard Medical School
Boston, MA

PROF. EVA BRAAK
Johann Wolfgang Goethe
  University
Department of Clinical
  Neuroanatomy
Frankfurt, GERMANY

DR. MED. HEIKO BRAAK
Johann Wolfgang Goethe
  University
Department of Clinical
  Neuroanatomy
Frankfurt, GERMANY

HERMAN BUSCHKE, M.D.
Albert Einstein College of
  Medicine
Bronx, NY

JEFFREY L. CUMMINGS,
  M.D.
Professor of Neurology and
  Psychiatry
David Geffen School of Medicine
  at UCLA
Los Angeles, CA

KELLY DEL TREDICI, PH.D.
Johann Wolfgang Goethe
  University
Department of Clinical
  Neuroanatomy
Frankfurt, GERMANY

TERESA GÓMEZ-ISLA, M.D.,
  PH.D.
Head of Memory Disorders
  Unit
Neurology Department
Clinica Universitaria de
  Navarra
Navarra, SPAIN

NEILL R. GRAFF-RADFORD,
   M.D.
Professor of Neurology
Mayo Medical School
Jacksonville, FL

BRADLEY T. HYMAN, M.D.,
   PH.D
Professor of Neurology
Massachusetts General Hospital
Harvard Medical School
Boston, MA

ROBERT J. IVNIK, PH.D.
Professor of Psychiatry and
   Psychology
Mayo Medical School
Rochester, MN

CLIFFORD R. JACK JR., M.D.
Professor of Radiology
Mayo Medical School
Rochester, MN

KEITH A. JOHNSON, M.D.
Assistant Professor of Neurology
Harvard Medical School
Boston, MA

DAVID S. KNOPMAN, M.D.
Professor of Neurology
Mayo Medical School
Rochester, MN

RICHARD LIPTON, M.D.
Albert Einstein College of
   Medicine
Bronx, NY

JOHN C. MORRIS, M.D.
Friedman Professor of Neurology
Washington University School of
   Medicine
St. Louis, MO

RONALD C. PETERSEN M.D.,
   PH.D.
Cora Kanow Professor of
   Alzheimer's Disease Research
Mayo Medical School
Rochester, MN

MARTIN SLIWINSKI, PH.D.
Department of Psychology
Syracuse University
Syracuse, NY

GLENN E. SMITH, PH.D.
Professor of Psychiatry and
   Psychology
Mayo Medical School
Rochester, MN

CHRISTINA WASYLYSHYN
Department of Psychology
Syracuse University
Syracuse, NY

MILD
COGNITIVE
IMPAIRMENT

CHAPTER **1**

Conceptual Overview

Ronald C. Petersen

Research in the field of aging and dementia is accelerating at an increasingly rapid rate. With the aging of America, the older segment of the population is increasing in size more rapidly than any other (Brookmeyer et al., 1998). People are living longer. In conjunction with this phenomenon comes concerns about the quality of life of persons as they age.

SCOPE OF THE PROBLEM

Dementia, and in particular Alzheimer's disease (AD), is a major concern for those individuals who live beyond the age of 70 years. While dementia is by no means a natural consequence of aging, both its incidence and its prevalence increase dramatically with age (Gao et al., 1998; Kukull and Ganguli, 2000). Consequently, a person aged 85 years has a one in three chance of having a significant cognitive impairment. Ultimately, as therapies progress, early identification may lead to prevention of age-related cognitive disabilities. All of this speaks to the importance of trying to identify cognitive impairment at its earliest stage.

These concerns about aging and cognitive impairment assume that we have a clear understanding of the border zone between normal aging and very early disease. While great strides have been made in recent decades in defining and characterizing dementia and AD, relatively less is known about the cognitive function in normal aging (Albert, 1997). Yet we presume we understand this aspect of cognition, since the definition of "abnormal" is predicated on the understanding of "normal."

As is depicted in Figure 1–1, there is likely a continuum between normal and abnormal function *in those subjects destined to develop dementia.* This is a theoretical model with many assumptions concerning the underlying dimensions, shape and slope of the curve. It should also be emphasized that this model *only* applies to those persons who are destined to develop dementia; it is not meant to represent an inevitable progression of cognitive change with age. It is quite likely that many elderly subjects can live successfully without any significant cognitive decline.

The clinical criteria for the diagnosis of probable AD have been well described (see Chapter 2), and the correspondences between the diagnosis of clinically probable AD and definite AD as determined by neuropathology criteria are quite high (Galasko et al., 1994). However, as can be seen in the figure, one phase of clinical impairment begins at the inflection point in the curve and precedes the point at which the subject meets the criteria for clinically probable AD. This region on the curve is

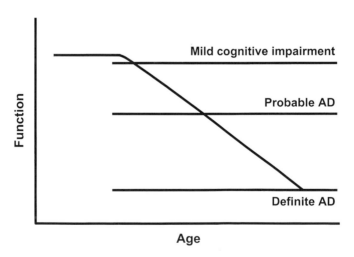

Figure 1–1. Theoretical continuum from normal aging through mild cognitive impairment to Alzheimer's disease. [Adapted from Petersen (2000), with permission.]

called *mild cognitive impairment* (*MCI*). During this phase, the sub-jects are experiencing subtle cognitive deficits with largely intact cognition and activities of daily living. The most frequent pre-sentation of this clinical condition is with forgetfulness. While there certainly can be other clinical presentations of MCI, as will be discussed later in this chapter, a subtle memory impairment is the most common initial complaint. Clinical criteria for MCI are shown in Table 1–1. As will be discussed in Chapter 2, this diagnosis is a clinical judgment, and while neuropsychological testing can be extremely useful, it is ultimately the judgment of the clinician that prevails in making this diagnosis.

As the literature on MCI expands, there is some confusion concerning the specific boundaries of the condition. There are several possible contributing factors to this inconsistency in the literature, such as clinical and etiological heterogeneity of the term, sources of study participants, reference points for normal aging, and use of rating scales. These will be discussed here.

HETEROGENEITY OF MILD COGNITIVE IMPAIRMENT

As the concept of MCI has become increasingly popular, impor-tant observations have been made about its definition, borders, and outcomes. At a conference on "Current Concepts in Mild Cognitive Impairment" in 1999 in Chicago, a group of experts from around the world convened and discussed issues concern-ing MCI (Petersen et al., 2001). There was consensus that MCI was an important topic of study but disagreement as to the uni-formity of its definition.

Mild cognitive impairment can be heterogeneous from two perspectives. From the first perspective, heterogeneity may refer to the *clinical presentation* of MCI (Petersen et al., 2001). As is

Table 1–1. Clinical Criteria for Mild Cognitive Impairment

1. Memory complaint, preferably corroborated by an informant
2. Objective memory impairment for age and education
3. Largely intact general cognitive function
4. Essentially preserved activities of daily living
5. Not demented

Source: Mayo Alzheimer Disease Center and Petersen et al. (1999).

shown in Figure 1–2, the *amnestic form of MCI* is most common, and most of the literature on the topic refers to this form of the disorder. In all likelihood, when this form of MCI is on a degenerative basis, the vast majority of cases will progress to AD. However, there may also be other clinical presentations of MCI. As is shown in Figure 1–2, another presentation could involve subjects being slightly impaired in multiple cognitive domains but not of sufficient magnitude to constitute dementia. This form, called *multiple-domain MCI*, may show a slight impairment in activities of daily living as well but, again, not of sufficient magnitude for the clinician to call the subject demented. To a certain extent, the concept of age-associated cognitive decline approximates this condition (Levy, 1994).

In the multiple-domain form of MCI, subjects may have a slight memory impairment in conjunction with mild impairments in, for example, executive function and language. The distinction between multiple-domain MCI and amnestic MCI is that no single domain is impaired out of proportion to the other cognitive domains. That is, in amnestic MCI, memory is affected to a significant degree—approximately 1.5 SD below age- and education-matched normal subjects—while other domains might be very mildly impaired at perhaps less than 0.5 SD below appropriate comparison subjects (Petersen et al., 1999). In multiple-domain MCI, several cognitive domains are impaired at perhaps the 0.5 to 1.0 SD level of impairment. (These ranges of

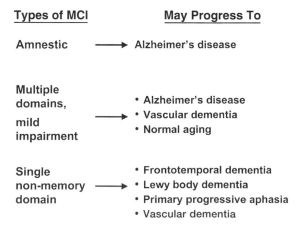

Figure 1–2. Clinical heterogeneity of mild cognitive impairment.

cognitive performance are only descriptive guidelines and do not imply specific cutoff scores.) The diagnosis of multiple-domain MCI is a clinical judgment on the part of the person evaluating the subject and cannot be made solely on the basis of neuro-psychological testing.

Persons with multiple-domain MCI may progress to AD or perhaps to vascular dementia. It is also possible that some of these subjects may represent an extreme of normal aging if they, in fact, do not progress and hence may be quite similar to what has been described as age-associated cognitive decline (Levy, 1994).

A third clinical variety of MCI could involve a mild impairment in a single non-memory cognitive domain. This form of MCI, known as *single non-memory-domain MCI* is characterized by a person having a relatively isolated impairment in a single non-memory domain such as executive function, visuospatial processing, or language. These mild conditions could represent incipient forms of other dementias. For example, the executive symptoms may lead to frontotemporal dementia (Rosen et al., 2000); a primary visuospatial impairment could lead to dementia with Lewy bodies (Ferman et al., 1999), or a prominent anomia might be the harbinger of primary progressive aphasia (Mesulam, 2001). Alternatively, any of these could lead to vascular dementia, depending on the specific location of the ischemia and the corresponding cognitive function that resides in that region (Chui, 2000). Conceptually it is quite likely that these other non-AD dementias have incipient stages, and while MCI may not be the best term for them, the terminology captures the concept of this prodromal state.

Figure 1–3 demonstrates the concept of incipient forms of a variety of dementias. It is likely as research progresses that the prodromal states of multiple conditions will become manifest, thus enabling intervention at an earlier state than is currently the practice.

In addition one can consider the *etiology* of the condition and the heterogeneity of causes. In its most common form, and the typical manner in which the term is used in the literature, MCI, particularly, amnestic MCI, is thought to evolve on a degenerative basis. This form of MCI presents with a memory impairment that gradually progresses to dementia and likely AD.

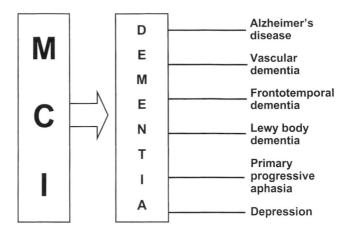

Figure 1–3. Mild cognitive impairment as a prodromal state for dementia that ultimately differentiates into a variety of clinical and pathological conditions.

While degeneration is the most common etiology, memory impairment could also evolve as a result of other conditions such as trauma, ischemia, depression, and substance abuse (e.g., alcohol), or there could be other non-AD degenerative causes as, for instance, hippocampal sclerosis. These non-AD causes may likely progress to other forms of dementia such as vascular dementia, or they may remain static and not progress. In fact, if there are false-positive diagnoses of patients with MCI who do not progress, these cases are likely due to other non-AD causes of the condition such as argyrophilic grain disease. Therefore, there can be heterogeneity in MCI due to the presumed etiology of the clinical condition.

To complicate matters, the two types of heterogeneity—etiology and clinical presentation—can be superimposed on each other. That is, these three types of clinical presentations—amnestic MCI, multiple-domain MCI, and single non-memory-domain MCI—may have multiple etiologies. As is shown in Figure 1–4, each clinical presentation could have a degenerative, vascular, metabolic, traumatic, or other causes. While this makes the classification of MCI somewhat complex, it also lends an element of organization to the overall conceptual scheme. These multiple layers of heterogeneity may also help explain some of the variability found in the scientific literature. At times the term

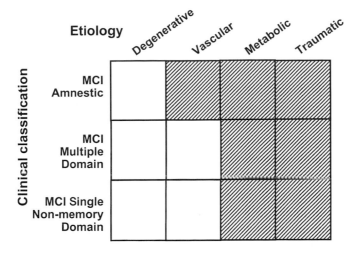

Figure 1–4. Heterogeneity of mild cognitive impairment from clinical and etiological perspectives. Open cells are most common.

"MCI" can be used quite loosely, which tends to confuse the underlying concept. Figure 1–4 is intended to present a theoretical framework from which to view the various concepts discussed here.

While these variations on the theme likely exist, by far the most common presentation of MCI is the amnestic type that is usually of a degenerative nature. As such, most of these subjects progress to AD, and this accounts for the bulk of the literature. These subjects have also become the intense study of multiple clinical trials (see Chapter 12).

SOURCES OF STUDY PARTICIPANTS

One source of variability among studies on MCI in the literature is derived from the recruitment strategies employed by the investigators. This factor can have a significant effect on the conclusions drawn from the study. Typically, subjects with a very mild degree of impairment such as that found in MCI often do not get referred to a dementia clinic for an evaluation. The subtle deficits that are found in these subjects are often overlooked by the subjects themselves, their families, and the examining physicians. If the study sample is derived primarily from subjects referred to a dementia or AD clinic, the subjects are likely to be more impaired than are individuals identified by community sampling. In addition, subjects who seek evaluation from a dementia clinic may be a "cleaner" group of individuals than those derived from a community-based setting. That is, when clinical and pathological studies are done on mild patients, the proportion of patients showing "pure" AD pathology is higher because of the inclusion criteria used to recruit subjects to these centers. This does not diminish the importance of the information gained from study of patients who present to clinics with memory impairment; rather, the derivation of patients is a source of variation that needs to be considered when interpreting the results.

An alternative to recruiting subjects from dementia clinics involves advertising in the mass media, but this strategy may also present problems. General advertising procedures can yield many responses and large numbers of individuals who may constitute "the worried well." An investigator may have to screen huge numbers of subjects with specially adapted instruments to yield a cohort of MCI subjects. This can be an effective strategy for identifying subjects, but careful attention needs to be paid to the screening process and the evaluation of the subjects (Daly et al., 2000).

Other proactive recruitment strategies can involve screening populations with a potential for high yield. By using appropriate techniques, investigators could survey geriatric clinics, general practice settings, or senior citizen activity centers. This strategy has the advantage of producing a higher yield of impaired persons because of the prevalence of cognitive disorders in this age group. It does not provide a population-based rate of impairment, however. Depending on the medical sophistication of the community, recruitment from primary care settings could be biased toward more affluent or health-conscious individuals.

Finally, investigators could conduct a population-based screening activity that is designed to evaluate elderly subjects sampled according to a prespecified scheme. In many respects, this is the optimal strategy, but it does have practical limitations. For example, if a large sample were to be studied, the evaluation must be somewhat abbreviated. It is difficult to use sufficiently sensitive instruments and an in-person clinical evaluation in this type of setting because they are expensive due to the magnitude of the sample. Unfortunately, since the diagnosis of MCI requires a significant degree of clinical sensitivity to early impairment, a thorough evaluation is difficult to perform on a large population-based sample. The time and expense involved in doing large-scale sampling exercises with thorough interviews and test batteries are problematical. In these settings, the quantity and perhaps the quality of the assessment may be compromised.

In general, there is no perfect study environment due to the limitations of recruitment, expenses, personnel, and the voluntary nature of the subject involvement in these research studies. This is not to say that each of these research contexts does not provide useful information; rather, investigators need to recognize the limitations of their own research settings and interpret the results accordingly.

REFERENCE POPULATIONS FOR NORMAL AGING

Persons with MCI have a memory impairment beyond what is expected for normal aging. Implicit in this definition is an understanding of what constitutes normal cognitive function with age. Unfortunately, this is not well understood. Most people believe that some loss of cognitive facility is a part of "normal" aging, while others contend that, in the absence of disease, there should be virtually no loss of function. As is typically the case, truth is somewhere in the middle. Most population-based studies of aging indicate that the vast majority of elderly subjects develop a decline in information processing speed and episodic memory function with age. These findings are sufficiently common that they must be accounted for in assessing departures from normal. The problem inherent in this issue concerns the selection of an appropriate normative standard against which to measure performance.

Some earlier studies have used performance of young adults as the standard, assuming that any differences found are due to the aging process (Crook et al., 1986). The difficulty with this approach is that, depending on which instruments are chosen, most of the elderly subjects will have "abnormal" performance when measured against younger adults (Smith et al., 1991).

Another approach involves the assessment of change in performance for a given individual over time (Collie and Maruff, 2000). This approach has the theoretical advantage of assessing performance on an individual subject basis, but the difficulties with this approach are twofold. First, from a practical standpoint, it is quite uncommon to have performance measures on individuals over a longitudinal period of time. Collie et al. (2001) argue that repeated assessments of psychomotor speed and memory over a relatively short period of time (months) establishes a baseline against which subsequent performance can be compared accurately. The value of this approach is yet to be validated longitudinally. Second, even with longitudinal data, it is not apparent what constitutes a meaningful change, especially in the very early stages of the MCI process. Consequently, while this approach certainly has its merit, the precise application of this strategy to practical clinical settings is not forthcoming immediately.

USE OF RATING SCALES

A source of confusion in the literature with respect to comparison of studies on MCI concerns the use of rating scales. Some studies define MCI using specific clinical criteria (see Chapter 2) (Petersen et al., 1999). Other studies equate cognitive stages on rating scales with MCI. For example, a popular rating scale for disease severity is the Clinical Dementia Rating scale (CDR) (Morris, 1993). The CDR can be employed using a semistructured interview that includes mental status components and emphasizes the importance of a knowledgeable informant. The CDR can also be used as a severity rating scale after a clinical diagnosis has been established by using standard criteria. It is not certain if the CDR scores derived in these two settings are equivalent. With this instrument, the summary score of CDR 0.5 has been believed to represent an intermediate stage of cognitive impairment or very mild dementia. In the early years in the use of this instrument, it is likely that the cases were felt to have "questionable dementia," as the stage was labeled. In more recent years, with improved sensitivity of the diagnosis of dementia, many CDR 0.5 cases have been classified clinically as having dementia (Morris et al., 2001). In fact, a controversy exists as to whether *all* CDR 0.5 subjects have dementia or more specifically AD while they are in this stage (Morris et al., 2001).

Investigators from Washington University contend that MCI is early AD since in their hands most CDR 0.5 subjects have pathological evidence of AD when they come to autopsy (Morris et al., 2001). However, most (approximately 70%) of the CDR 0.5 subjects at Washington University also have the clinical diagnosis of AD at the CDR 0.5 stage. They contend that their CDR 0.5 "incipient AD" subjects are equivalent to MCI subjects at other institutions. However, all of their subjects whom they designate as incipient AD have been diagnosed by them as having clinically probable AD. As such, since the MCI clinical criteria preclude the diagnosis of dementia or AD, these subjects cannot be the same as MCI subjects diagnosed elsewhere. The Washington University investigators do not have a clinical classification equivalent to MCI in their diagnostic system. These investigators believe that other clinicians are likely "undercalling" these subjects as having MCI when they actually are demented. This remains a topic of investigation.

Therefore, while all MCI subjects who fulfill clinical criteria are also likely to have CDR 0.5, the converse is not necessarily true: that is, some CDR 0.5 subjects may have MCI, and some may have dementia. The CDR 0.5 classification is not identical to the clinical classification of MCI.

In a similar vein, the Global Deterioration Scale (GDS) has been used to classify the severity of normal and demented subjects (Reisberg et al., 1982). The GDS ranges from 1 (normal) to 2 (normal with a subjective complaint) on to stages 3 through 7, which represent increasing levels of impairment. Investigators at New York University contend that the GDS of 3 is equivalent to MCI as defined by other investigators using clinical criteria (Kluger et al., 1999). In a fashion similar to the use of the CDR, subjects with a GDS of 3 may have MCI or may be mildly demented (Flicker et al., 1991). In the Mayo Clinic series of MCI subjects, the mean GDS for subjects classified with MCI by clinical criteria was 2.7, indicating that some have the classification of GDS 2 and some GDS 3 (Petersen et al., 1999). The GDS ratings from a large multicenter treatment trial for MCI sponsored by the National Institute on Aging through the Alzheimer's Disease Cooperative Study was also in the 2.7 range. Therefore, no single GDS stage maps directly onto the MCI subjects when clinical criteria are used to classify them.

In summary, rating scales are very useful for staging subjects, but they do not necessarily provide criteria for characterizing

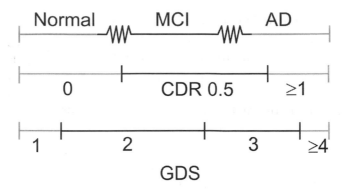

Figure 1–5. Lack of direct correspondence between Clinical Dementia Rating (CDR) scale 0.5, Global Deterioration Scale (GDS) stage 3, and clinical definition of mild cognitive impairment. [Adapted from Petersen (2000), with permission.]

subjects with MCI as outlined in Table 1–1. As is depicted in Figure 1–5, the reader of the literature needs to be aware of the precise manner in which the subjects in an MCI study are characterized. If the definition involves a single stage on a rating scale, the subjects may be more heterogeneous with respect to level of severity than if the subjects are defined on the basis of clinical criteria.

FUTURE DIRECTIONS

Ultimately, MCI is likely to be a heuristic concept. It has generated and will continue to spawn research on aging and early cognitive impairment. At some point, the term will be discarded, and another will take its place. Hopefully, the concept will have contributed to an understanding of the spectrum of cognition from normal aging to AD.

It is likely that the threshold for the clinical diagnosis of AD may be moved back to encompass milder forms of impairment and possibly MCI. Alternatively, MCI may continue to occupy a niche in the cognitive spectrum that cannot be subsumed by other clinical classifications; it may truly be a transitional stage in the development of AD. Additional neuropathological data may shed light on this issue when they are available from a variety of clinical settings. It is likely that some subjects with MCI harbor the early features of evolving AD, but probably not all of them do. Other subjects may have other non-AD pathological features of medial temporal lobe damage.

To a certain extent, the challenge in the field revolves around certain semantic (definitional) issues. For example, what is normal aging? How do you define "normal"? Is it statistically normal, ideally normal, or typically normal? This is not well delineated. Without a definite biomarker, then, at what point do you state that a person has AD? Is it when they reach a clinical threshold of impairment, or is it when they possess any neuropathologic features of AD in the brain? Does the presence of pathological features of AD in the brain necessarily mean that the individual will progress to dementia? Can these pathological features be detected by new imaging techniques? These are difficult questions at present, but future investigations may help clarify them.

This book will attempt to address these issues. The authors were asked to address the questions of the threshold between aging and very mild impairment from their own perspectives. As you will see, there can be diverse opinions on these questions, and we hope the ensuing discussions will stimulate further research and insight into these important issues.

References

Albert, M.S. (1997). The ageing brain: normal and abnormal memory. *Phil Trans Royal Soc London—Series B: Biol Sci* 352:1703–1709.

Brookmeyer, R., S. Gray, and C. Kawas. (1998). Projections of Alzheimer's disease in the United States and the public health impact of delaying disease onset. *Am J Pub Health* 88:1337–1342.

Chui, H. (2000). Vascular dementia, a new beginning: shifting focus from clinical phenotype to ischemic brain injury. *Neurol Clin* 18:951–978.

Collie, A., and P. Maruff. (2000). The neuropsychology of preclinical Alzheimer's disease and mild cognitive impairment. *Neurosci Biobehav Rev* 24(3):365–374.

Collie, A., P. Maruff, R. Shafiq-Antonacci, M. Smith, M. Hallup, P.R. Schofield, C.L. Masters, and J. Currie. (2001). Memory decline in healthy older people: implications for identifying mild cognitive impairment. *Neurology* 56:1533–1538.

Crook, T., R.T. Bartus, S.H. Ferris, P. Whitehouse, G.D. Cohen, and S. Gershon. (1986). Age-associated memory impairment: proposed diagnostic criteria and measures of clinical change—report of a National Institute of Mental Health Work Group. *Devel Neuropsychol* 2:261–276.

Daly, E., D. Zaitchik, M. Copeland, J. Schmahmann, J. Gunther, and M. Albert. (2000). Predicting conversion to Alzheimer's disease using standardized clinical information. *Arch Neurol* 57(5):675–680.

Ferman, T.J., B.F. Boeve, G.E. Smith, M.H. Silber, E. Kokmen, R.C. Petersen, and R.J. Ivnik. (1999). REM sleep behavior disorder and dementia: cognitive differences when compared with AD. *Neurology* 52:951–957.

Flicker, C., S.H. Ferris, and B. Reisberg. (1991). Mild cognitive impairment in the elderly: predictors of dementia. *Neurology* 41:1006–1009.

Galasko, D., L.A. Hansen, R. Katzman, W. Wiederholt, E. Masliah, R. Terry, L.R. Hill, P. Lessin, and L.J. Thal. (1994). Clinical-neuropathological correlations in Alzheimer's disease and related dementias. *Arch Neurol* 51:888–895.

Gao, S., H.C. Hendrie, K.S. Hall, and S. Hui. (1998). The relationship between age, sex, and the incidence of dementia and Alzheimer disease: a meta-analysis. *Arch Gen Psychiatry* 55:809–815.

Kluger, A., S.H. Ferris, J. Golomb, M.S. Mittelman, and B. Reisberg. (1999). Neuropsychological prediction of decline to dementia in nondemented elderly. *J Geriatr Psychiatry Neurol* 12:168–179.

Kukull, W.A., and M. Ganguli. (2000). Epidemiology of dementia: concepts and overview. In Neurologic Clinics, edited by S. DeKosky. Philadelphia: W.B. Saunders.

Levy, R. (1994). Aging-associated cognitive decline. *Int Psychogeriatr* 6:63–68.

Mesulam, M-Marsel. (2001). Primary progressive aphasia. *Ann Neurol* 49:425–432.

Morris, J.C. (1993). The Clinical Dementia Rating (CDR): current version and scoring rules. *Neurology* 43:2412–2414.

Morris, J.C., M. Storandt, J.P. Miller, D.W. McKeel, J.L. Price, E.H. Rubin, and L. Berg. (2001). Mild cognitive impairment represents early-stage Alzheimer's disease. *Arch Neurol* 58:397–405.

Petersen, R.C., G.E. Smith, S.C. Waring, R.J. Ivnik, E.G. Tangalos, and E. Kokmen. (1999). Mild cognitive impairment: clinical characterization and outcome. *Arch Neurol* 56:303–308.

Petersen, R.C. (2000). Aging, mild cognitive impairment, and Alzheimer's disease. In Neurologic Clinics, edited by S. DeKosky. Philadelphia: W.B. Saunders.

Petersen, R.C., R. Doody, A. Kurz, R.C. Mohs, J.C. Morris, P.V. Rabins, K. Ritchie, M. Rossor, L. Thal, and B. Winblad. (2001). Current concepts in mild cognitive impairment. *Arch Neurol* 58:1985–1992.

Reisberg, B., S.H. Ferris, M.J. de Leon, and T. Crook. (1982). The Global Deterioration Scale for assessment of primary degenerative dementia. *Am J Psychiatry* 139:1136–1139.

Rosen, H.J., J. Lengenfelder, and B. Miller. (2000). Frontotemporal dementia. In Neurologic Clinics, edited by S.T. DeKosky. Philadelphia: W.B. Saunders.

Smith, G., R.J. Ivnik, R.C. Petersen, J.F. Malec, E. Kokmen, and E. Tangalos. (1991). Age-associated memory impairment diagnoses: problems of reliability and concerns for terminology. *Psychol Aging* 6(4):551–558.

CHAPTER **2**

Clinical Features

RONALD C. PETERSEN
JOHN C. MORRIS

It has become increasingly evident in recent years that prodromal states of Alzheimer's disease (AD) likely exist. Clinical criteria for AD have been published and used worldwide—for example, *Diagnostic and Statistical Manual IV* (*DSM IV*) and National Institute for Neurological Communitive Disorders and Stroke/Alzheimer's Disease and Related Disorders (NINCDS/ADRDA) (*Diagnostic and Statistical Manual of Mental Disorders*, 4th ed., 1994; McKhann et al., 1984). These have been very useful, but they are designed to detect the disease in the reasonably well developed state: that is, the criteria require impairments in memory and other cognitive domains of sufficient severity to affect functional activities. Persons must have multiple cognitive and functional impairments to qualify for this diagnosis. These criteria have performed very well for their intended purposes.

Recent research has indicated, however, that there is likely a phase of cognitive impairment before a person reaches full criteria for AD (Petersen, 2000a). This intermediate stage has been referred to by various names, including incipient dementia, prodromal AD, isolated memory impairment, and—as it will be labeled in this discussion—mild cognitive impairment (MCI) (Tierney et al., 1996; Bowen et al., 1997; Petersen et al., 1999;

Daly et al., 2000; Bozoki et al., 2001). Figure 2–1 depicts a theoretical continuum of progression from normal aging through MCI to probable AD and definite AD (Petersen, 1995). It is important to note that this framework is not a model of aging in general; rather, it depicts the hypothetical course of progression in persons who are destined to develop AD.

As the figure indicates, there is an overlap in the boundaries between normal aging and MCI, and between MCI and AD. These boundaries represent challenges for investigators studying this area.

HISTORY

The concept of a memory impairment developing with aging has been discussed in the literature for many years. Perhaps the first discussion of this type of problem was introduced by Kral (1962) with his term, "benign senescent forgetfulness." This term referred to memory changes that were likely relatively stable and not indicative of a progressive disorder. Typically, these persons had difficulties with recall of details of events but were not experiencing major forgetfulness. Kral suggested that individuals with benign senescent forgetfulness did not tend to progress to dementia.

In 1986, the National Institute of Mental Health organized a workgroup to address cognitive changes with age and coined

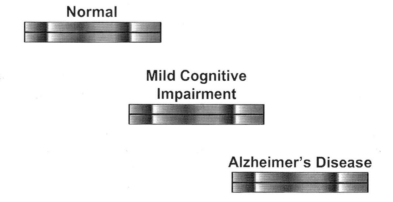

Figure 2–1. Theoretical transitional states from normal aging through mild cognitive impairment to Alzheimer's disease. [Adapted from Petersen (1995), with permission.]

the term, "age-associated memory impairment" (AAMI) (Crook et al., 1986). This concept generated a great deal of research and moved the field forward. Criteria for this concept included a subjective memory impairment, normal general cognition, no dementia, and an objective memory impairment 1 SD below that of young adults. The last criterion produced difficulty for the concept because individual memory tests were not specified by the workgroup. Depending on which particular memory test was to be used, virtually all older individuals may qualify for the diagnosis of AAMI. For example, Smith and colleagues (1991) demonstrated that using a difficult memory test such as the Auditory Verbal Learning Test and using the measure of delayed recall, 90% of otherwise normal elderly subjects would qualify for AAMI. Although the AAMI concept stimulated a great deal of research on memory and aging, the usefulness of this construct as defined was questioned.

Levy (1994) and colleagues with the International Psychogeriatric Association proposed a revision of the AAMI construct with the notion of "aging-associated cognitive decline" (AACD). This concept broadened the notion of impairment to domains other than memory. Persons with AACD may have deficits in memory, attention, language, or visuospatial skills, and performance was referenced to age-appropriate norms. The deficits were not believed to be sufficiently severe to impair functional activities. The criteria for AACD refer to a person who is aware of a cognitive decline for at least 6 months and has objective evidence of a cognitive decline in learning, memory, attention, thinking, language, and visuospatial skills of a magnitude of at least 1 SD below age and education norms. It is not certain if this concept refers to a manifestation of normal aging or incipient disease. This issue may relate to alternative types of MCI.

The *DSM IV* has addressed cognitive changes with age in the research nomenclature in the manual and proposed the term, "aging-related cognitive decline" (*Diagnostic and Statistical Manual of Mental Disorders*, 4th ed., 1994). This term is meant to refer to cognitive changes resulting from the aging process, such as a change in memory or other cognitive process not believed to be related to neurologic or psychiatric disorders. However, this concept was somewhat vague and did not address the issue of normal aging and incipient disease.

The International Classification of Disease 10 (ICD 10) proposed the concept of a mild cognitive disorder, which referred to an impairment of memory or concentration that was not believed to be due to dementia or other nervous system disorders but, rather, to systemic illnesses. In this sense, the concept is only tangentially related to the notion of MCI.

Finally, the Canadian Study of Health and Aging developed the concept of "cognitive impairment—no dementia" (Graham et al., 1997) This broad term likely encompasses MCI as it is defined here, but it also refers to other nonprogressive entities such as static encephalopathies. While some individuals in this category would qualify for MCI, others may have a delirium, alcoholism, or a static process such as mental retardation. Still other individuals in this classification scheme would qualify for MCI but would need to be isolated by a separate set of criteria. Recent subdivisions of this classification have identified subgroups that may approximate MCI. Nevertheless, the longitudinal follow-up of persons in the Canadian Study of Health and Aging should provide useful information on persons with MCI.

CLINICAL STUDIES AND OUTCOMES

Mayo Clinic

The Mayo Clinic research group has been following a group of subjects aging in the community of Rochester, Minnesota, for over 15 years (Petersen et al., 1990). This study of aging and dementia has enrolled subjects who have had any degree of cognitive impairment and also enrolled a group of age- and gender-matched control subjects. The entire cohort is followed longitudinally on an annual basis. Over the years this project has enrolled over 1900 subjects. The recruitment mechanism is unique, but important, for the accrual of mildly impaired subjects.

Many of the residents of Rochester, Minnesota, receive their general medical care from primary care physicians at the Mayo Clinic. As such, the research staff reviews the medical histories of all persons aged 65 years and over who have received a general medical examination. If in this review there is any mention of a cognitive issue—for example, "I have been having trouble with names" or "My husband is more forgetful"—or if the physician comments on the patient's cognitive status, the staff notes this, and the primary care physician is contacted for permission to enroll the subject in the research project. This mechanism results in a number of false positives—those subjects who casually mention a cognitive concern to their physician but who are functioning quite normally. However, it also allows the research group to recruit subjects at the very earliest point in their cognitive impairment. This is an active recruitment strategy that is designed to detect early cognitive impairment rather than waiting for subjects to be passively referred by themselves, family, or physicians. The latter procedure often results in referrals being delayed until the person is more advanced in their cognitive impairment.

This recruitment strategy has yielded subjects with MCI from two sources. One source is as described above, which is derived from the general medical examinations performed by the primary care physicians. The other group is derived from the longitudinal follow-up of the normal control subjects. Over the years, more than 70 formerly normal subjects have evolved to MCI status.

Subjects who have been followed in Rochester, Minnesota, have been the source of numerous studies of normal cognition and have provided data for normative neuropsychology work (see Chapter 5) (Ivnik et al., 1992, 1994, 1995, 1999; Smith et al., 1992, 1994a, 1994b, 1997). This work provides the necessary background for judging normal cognitive function against whom the mild cognitive impairment subjects can be compared.

The criteria that have been used for MCI by the Mayo Clinic research group include the following:

• Memory complaint, preferably corroborated by an informant
• Objective memory impairment for age and education
• Largely normal general cognitive function
• Essentially intact activities of daily living
• Not demented

The challenge for the field revolves around the operationalization of these criteria. It must be emphasized that the criteria are *clinical*. That is, the criteria are employed during a consensus meeting involving behavioral neurologists, neuropsychologists, a

geriatrician, and nurses who have evaluated the subjects in a fashion similar to that used to make the diagnosis of dementia or
AD. In general, the criteria are satisfied as follows.

The subjective memory complaint is elicited from the subjects and preferably from an informant who knows the subject
well. However, 40% of the subjects in the Mayo research studies
live alone, so a close informant may not be available. As is well
known in the literature, subjects' memory complaints are of variable reliability. In some instances they connote an affective state
(Bassett and Folstein, 1993; Tobiansky et al., 1995; Ritchie et al.,
1996; Smith et al., 1996; Dartigues et al., 1997; Schofield et al.,
1997a; Riedel-Heller et al., 1999). However, in some instances
these complaints can actually portend a subsequent cognitive decline (O'Brien et al., 1992; Tobiansky et al., 1995; Schmand et
al., 1996; Dartigues et al., 1997; Schofield et al., 1997b; Geerlings
et al., 1999). An important adjunct, if available, is corroboration
by an informant (Tierney et al., 1996). This piece of information
can be very helpful.

The objective memory impairment has caused some confusion in the recent literature. As discussed here, the diagnosis of
MCI by the Mayo group is clinical. The memory impairment is
a clinical judgment based on the subject's history, the clinician's
examination, and the neuropsychological profile. Memory function is usually assessed by learning over trials or delayed recall
on a multiple-trial free-recall task such as the Auditory Verbal
Learning Test or, possibly, the Wechsler Memory Scale–Revised
or III, Logical Memory II, or Visual Reproduction II (Rey, 1964;
Wechsler, 1987). There are no cutoff scores on any neuropsychological test; rather, the profile of memory function being impaired out of proportion to tests of other cognitive domains is
most important. In general, when the MCI subjects' memory performances on the delayed recall measures are assessed as a
group, the subjects tend to fall 1.5 SD below age- and education-
matched subjects from the Mayo normative data sample (Petersen et al., 1999). However, it must be emphasized that this level
of performance is not used as a cutoff score. In fact, there is a
range of performance around the mean.

In a similar fashion, the criterion of normal general cognitive function involves a clinical judgment. The non-memory cognitive domains of attention, language, visuospatial function,
problem solving, and the like are not impaired to a sufficient

extent to lead the clinician to believe that they are significantly impaired; that is, meeting criteria for dementia. Some of the domains are statistically significantly reduced relative to control subjects, but generally this difference is only of the magnitude of approximately 0.5 SD or less. Again, this figure is derived from group data and does not constitute a cutoff score.

The next criterion refers to generally intact activities of daily living. Most of this information is derived from a history taken from the subject and informant and is documented using the Record of Independent Living and Clinical Dementia Rating (Weintraub, 1986; Morris, 1993; Smith et al., 2000). Once again, this involves the judgment of the clinician and can be quite challenging. Often these persons have experienced some change in their lifestyle over the years, but the clinician must decide if the changes are due to an alteration in cognition or to other physical problems and conditions. In addition, the clinician must discern if the changes are of sufficient magnitude to constitute evidence for dementia.

Finally, and perhaps most important, in the judgment of the clinician, the subject does not meet criteria for dementia. That is, after the memory changes are evaluated, general cognition is assessed, and activities of daily living are evaluated with the informant, the clinician does not believe that the subject meets standard criteria (*DSM III-R*, or *DSM IV* for dementia and NINCDS-ADRDA for AD). This is becoming increasingly challenging as the threshold for determining dementia moves increasingly toward milder degrees of impairment.

Over 15 years the Mayo research group has evaluated more than 270 individuals who have fulfilled clinical criteria for MCI. When characterized in this fashion, they tend to progress to dementia or clinically probable AD at a rate of 10% to 15% per year (Petersen et al., 1999). Most recently, the figures have approximated 12% per year. This is in contrast to the normal control cohort in Rochester, which develops MCI/AD at a rate of 1% to 2% per year (Petersen et al., 1999). Figure 2–2 demonstrates the data presented as a survival curve, indicating that after approximately 6 years, 80% of the MCI cohort has declined to dementia.

It is likely that not all of these subjects will ultimately decline to dementia or AD. The final numbers may extend to the range of 80% to 90%. The residual 10% (or more) will possibly include

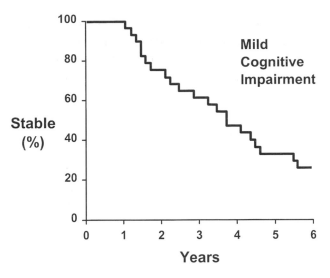

Figure 2–2. Survival curve showing proportion of individuals who remain in the state of mild cognitive impairment through succeeding years. [Adapted from Petersen et al. (2001), with permission.]

persons with other processes that affect medial temporal lobe structures, such as hippocampal sclerosis or trauma. There also may be some individuals who have had a lifelong tendency to be "slow learners" and now are experiencing changes of aging and hence appear to meet criteria for MCI but, in fact, are not progressing to dementia. However, the vast majority of the subjects when characterized as amnestic MCI go on to develop clinically probable AD. As such, MCI defined in this fashion is a prodromal, at-risk condition for AD.

Washington University

The Washington University cohort is a convenience sample of elderly individuals recruited from the greater St. Louis area by media appeals, physician referrals, and "word of mouth" to participate in longitudinal studies of healthy aging and dementia. Enrollment was initiated in 1979; all participants are evaluated annually with standard clinical and psychometric assessments. All assessments are for research purposes only (i.e., medical management is not provided). Dementia diagnosis is based on the clinical assessment of the individual and on a semistructured interview with a collateral source (typically the spouse or adult child) and is made without reference to psychometric performance or scores on cognitive tests such as the Mini-Mental State Examination (MMSE) (Folstein et al., 1975). The interview does include some mental status assessment items such as a recall of a short phrase.

Information from the collateral source is sought to ascertain whether the individual has experienced memory and other cognitive deficits that represent a decline from a previous level of cognitive function and whether the deficits compromise the individual's ability to carry out their usual activities in the community, at home, and in social relationships. The collateral source typically is able to observe whether activities such as driving a motor vehicle, shopping, cooking, handling finances, effecting home repairs, or participating in card games or other hobbies are conducted less well by the individual, even if still being performed, because of cognitive loss. That is, the collateral source–based clinical assessment is sensitive to even mild interference in the individual's capacity to conduct everyday activities and thus often is more sensitive to early-stage dementia than is cognitive test performance (Morris et al., 1996) or the self-report of the individual (Carr et al., 2000). The collateral source–based method is especially important for individuals who have superior baseline intellectual function and who still score in the normal range on cognitive measures in spite of mild dementia.

Dementia staging at Washington University is conducted independently of psychometric testing and is based solely on the clinical assessment. A Clinical Dementia Rating (CDR) is assigned such that CDR 0 indicates no dementia and CDR 0.5, 1, 2, and 3 indicate very mild, mild, moderate, and severe dementia (Morris, 1993; Morris et al., 1993). The clinical diagnosis of dementia of the Alzheimer type (DAT) is in accordance with standard criteria and is confirmed by the neuropathologic presence of AD and autopsy in 93% of cases (Berg et al., 1998).

Nondemented individuals in this sample maintain their cognitive performance over time. In 82 individuals who entered in the CDR 0 stage, 60% ($n = 55$) remained at CDR 0 up to 15 years later. Of these 55 nondemented individuals, 48 showed no decline in annual psychometric performance (represented by a standardized factor score indicating general cognitive ability) (Rubin et al., 1998). Although learning effects and acclimation to repeated testing might offset mild decrements in performance associated with age, nonetheless these data suggest that substantial cognitive decline is not part of truly healthy brain aging. When cognitive deficits do occur, therefore, they may represent the onset of dementing illness rather than a "benign" aspect of aging. Indeed, data from this cohort suggest that individuals who meet criteria for AAMI are at substantially greater risk for developing overt dementia than are individuals who do not have AAMI (Goldman and Morris, 2001).

To address whether "MCI-equivalent individuals" may already manifest the initial clinical manifestations of AD (rather than a "normal" consequence of aging), all individuals with an initial designation of CDR 0.5 were classified into three categories. There were 105 individuals (mean age = 76 years; mean MMSE score = 24) who were believed to already have DAT (CDR 0.5/DAT); 69 individuals (mean age = 78 years; mean MMSE score = 26) who were believed to have incipient DAT but who were given the clinical diagnosis of very mild DAT (CDR 0.5/incipient); and 53 individuals (mean age = 76 years; mean MMSE score = 29) with uncertain dementia (CDR 0.5/uncertain). Over 5 years, progression to greater dementia severity (CDR 1 or greater) occurred in 60% of CDR 0.5/DAT, 36% of CDR 0.5/incipient, and 20% of CDR 0.5/uncertain individuals; only 7% of CDR 0 individuals progressed to CDR 1 or greater stage over this period (Morris et al., 2001). Extending the period of observation to 9.5 years found that all surviving CDR 0.5/DAT individuals had progressed to AD. All 32 individuals who came to autopsy (including 8 CDR 0.5/incipient (2 of whom remainded incipient at death) and 6 CDR 0.5/uncertain cases) had a neuropathologic dementing illness, and 28 (88%) of them had AD (Morris et al., 2001). In contrast, 9 of the 10 CDR 0 individuals studied postmortem had lacked neuropathologic AD (Morris et al., 2001).

The Washington University group believes that their CDR 0.5 incipient AD subjects are similar to what is described elsewhere as amnestic MCI. One difference is related to the clinical diagnosis of probable AD: other investigators do not feel the amnestic MCI subjects are demented, while the Washington University group classifies their subjects as probable AD. It is not certain if these subjects are similar. For those CDR 0.5 individuals (i.e., CDR 0.5/incipient) who resemble the amnestic MCI category discussed above and even for CDR 0.5 individuals (i.e., CDR 0.5/uncertain) less impaired than MCI, there is predictable progression to greater stages of dementia. The rate of progression varies with the level of impairment at baseline, so that the less the severity, the slower the rate of progression. The CDR 0.5/ incipient and CDR 0.5/uncertain individuals are less impaired than the CDR 0.5/DAT individuals and hence progress more slowly; periods of observation even longer than 9 years may be required to determine progression in these less-impaired groups. The neuropathology of CDR 0.5 in this sample overwhelmingly is AD at Washington University. As validated by clinical course (progression to greater dementia severity) and by autopsy findings of AD, CDR 0.5 appears to represent the earliest symptomatic stage of AD. The detection of this very mild stage of AD depends on collateral source–based clinical assessment methods rather than on psychometric performance. It appears that DAT can be diagnosed at earlier stages than currently is practiced.

Toronto

Tierney and colleagues (1996a, 1996b) from Toronto have evaluated a cohort of subjects referred from family practitioners who had memory impairment but did not meet the criteria for dementia. Over the course of 2 years, 107 subjects were followed and 29 developed AD while 78 did not (13.5% per year). This was a prospective study, including subjects who were evaluated by an experienced clinician, and causes of memory impairment other than a degenerative nature were excluded. Patients meeting criteria for dementia using *DSM III-R* criteria at the outset were excluded. Subjects were administered neuropsychological tests, but the clinician and the neuropsychologist assessed the patients independently. In this sense, this experience closely resembles the Mayo Clinic and Washington University data already reported here.

Seattle

Bowen and colleagues (1997) from an HMO in Seattle followed a registry of 811 patients with cognitive complaints for a mean of 48 months. They identified 21 patients with an isolated memory loss of unknown cause and compared them to a group of 198 subjects from the same source with newly recognized cognitive complaints but no dementia or memory loss. Over the follow-up, 10 (48%) of the memory loss subjects and 36 (18%) of the comparison group developed dementia. These data, while involving small numbers of subjects show a progression rate of 12% per year.

Massachusetts General Hospital

Albert and colleagues (Daly et al., 2000) at the Massachusetts General Hospital have established a longitudinal study of subjects characterized as having "questionable dementia" meeting CDR 0.5 criteria. These investigators used a university-based program setting to recruit cognitively impaired subjects through advertising in the media. They screened participants using a modification of the CDR and followed subjects for 3 years. During this time period, 23 of the 123 subjects (6% per year) with a questionable dementia converted to probable AD. This conversion rate is lower than others reported in the literature, which characterize subjects with an intermediate degree of cognitive impairment. This may be due to several factors, including the source of the subjects obtained through media advertising and perhaps to a higher education level of the subjects in this population. This study emphasizes the importance of a detailed history obtained for the purpose of detecting an early cognitive impairment.

Montpellier, France

Ritchie and colleagues (2000) have recently reported a study designed to compare MCI criteria with age-associated cognitive decline (AACD). The study retrospectively fit neuropsychologically based criteria for MCI to a group of subjects from a sample of general practitioners. The subjects were normal at enrollment and were followed for 3 years. Some 833 subjects older than 60 years of age were enrolled and were sent a proxy screening questionnaire to assess changes in cognitive function over the previous years. The proxy had to have monthly contact with the subject over a 3-year period. Using this instrument, 397 subjects showed some cognitive decline and had subjective complaints. These subjects were compared to a random sample of 73 who did not have cognitive complaints. All 833 subjects were also given a computerized neuropsychological examination. The subjects were evaluated with a neurologic examination only in the third year. The investigators applied a modification of the Mayo Clinic criteria retrospectively to this sample. The deviations from the Mayo application of the criteria were significant. For a memory impairment, the investigators applied a criterion of 1 SD on their memory task, which included recall of names and faces. They interpreted the criterion of a normal general cognitive function as estimated by performance on a vocabulary test. The subjects had to be at or above the mean for their reference group. (This criterion is not used by Mayo researchers.) The operationalization of the AACD criteria was not given.

When the modifications of the MCI criteria were used, they found only 27 persons of their group of 397 subjects met their criteria for MCI, while 174 were classified with AACD. Following these subjects over 3 years demonstrated that this definition of MCI was unstable, while the AACD criteria appeared to have better prediction for dementia.

These data are difficult to interpret when compared to the other studies assessing the concept of MCI. The criteria were unique to this study and did not correspond to the definition of MCI proposed in other studies. This study constituted a retrospective fit of neuropsychological criteria to a database. Consequently, this approach deviated from the clinical procedures used to make the diagnosis of MCI by Mayo researchers and in other prospective longitudinal studies. The Mayo data indicated that while memory is impaired out of proportion to other cognitive domains, other cognitive functions are also slightly impaired. Therefore, the literal interpretation of MCI criteria as done in this French study were not comparable. Experienced clinicians need to be involved in the diagnostic process to ensure consistency in the application of the criteria.

Interestingly, while AACD was conceived as a variation of normal, this study indicated that several of the persons designated with AACD actually went on to develop dementia. Although these investigators concluded that MCI is unstable, their interpretation was flawed because of the application of unique criteria that did not allow for comparisons with other studies. While AACD was conceived as a variation of normal, this study indicated that a substantial proportion of the persons designated with AACD actually went on to develop dementia. Nevertheless, this study was useful in demonstrating that variable outcomes in subjects designated with MCI can be found, depending on the application of various criteria.

New York University

The research group at New York University (NYU) was one of the first to use the term, "mild cognitive impairment" (Flicker et al., 1991). Essentially, these investigators defined MCI using the Global Deterioration Scale (GDS) (Reisberg et al., 1982). In a recent review of this work by Kluger et al. (1999), longitudinal data using the GDS were summarized. One of the first studies addressing this issue by Flicker and colleagues (1991) followed 32 GDS 1–2 subjects and 32 GDS 3 subjects for 2 years; over this time span, they observed that 72% of the GDS 3 subjects progressed to dementia and about 50% of them to AD. However, those GDS subjects who progressed had deficits in verbal recall, visuospatial recall, and certain aspects of language function at baseline, raising the suspicion that these GDS 3 subjects may be more impaired at the outset than were the subjects defined with MCI criteria by other research groups.

The NYU group has characterized normal subjects as having a GDS 1 or 2. The GDS 2 subjects are normal but have a subjective impression of a memory impairment. Interestingly, however, their data indicate that while none of the GDS 1 subjects declined on an annual basis, approximately 3.7% of the GDS 2 subjects declined (Kluger et al., 1999). The 0% rate is unusual since in a typical elderly population, dementia incidence rates are between 1% and 2% per year. This may suggest that the GDS 1 control subjects in this study are particularly healthy. In contrast, the GDS 2 group's annual conversion rate is high for control subjects, implying that there may be some MCI subjects in the GDS 2 category. The GDS 3 subjects appear to progress to GDS 4 at a reasonably high rate, again implying that this group may include both MCI subjects and mildly demented subjects. Consequently, like the CDR, the GDS only approximates MCI, and no single rating stage corresponds perfectly with the Mayo amnestic MCI criteria outlined earlier (Petersen et al., 1999).

Columbia University

Devanand and colleagues (1997, 2000) at Columbia University have been particularly interested in studying olfaction in MCI.

They have reported a group of 99 MCI subjects, 77 of whom were followed for 2 years. They defined MCI as a CDR of 0 or 0.5 and an equivalent MMSE score of 22 or greater. They used neuro-psychological testing guidelines such as fewer than 3/3 recall on the modified MMSE at 5 minutes and an impaired delayed recall score greater than 1 SD below norms on the Selective Remind-ing Test or impaired Wechsler Adult Intelligence Scale–R Per-formance IQ of greater than or equal to 10 points below the Verbal IQ. The neuropsychological guidelines were used as ref-erences since the final diagnosis was made by two expert clini-cians. The diagnosis of dementia was made by *DSM IV* criteria and possible and probable AD by NINCDS-ADRDA criteria (*Di-agnostic and Statistical Manual of Mental Disorders*, 4th ed., 1994; McKhann et al., 1984). Using this procedure, they found that approximately 12.3% of the MCI subjects progressed to AD per year. This clinic-based experience matched other community-based series quite closely.

University of Michigan

Investigators at the University of Michigan have identified ret-rospectively a group of 48 subjects whom they have labeled as having an isolated memory impairment (Bozoki et al., 2001). They further subdivided these subjects into those who had a rel-atively pure memory deficit and those who had a memory deficit plus slight impairments in other cognitive domains. However, none of these impairments was of sufficient magnitude to con-stitute the diagnosis of dementia. They found that those subjects with additional cognitive domains impaired progressed more rap-idly to dementia (24% per year) than those with just a memory impairment (3% per year). These results are quite similar to other studies on MCI insofar as a group of nondemented but cognitively impaired subjects were identifiable, and those with more significant cognitive impairments tended to progress more rapidly.

Bordeaux, France

A research team from Bordeaux has been following a community-based cohort of 3777 subjects from two areas in southwestern France; they recently reported incidence figures for MCI (Lar-rieu et al., in press). This study is different from the Montpellier,

France, study just discussed in that a neurologist evaluated these subjects initially and at each follow-up assessment and rated the subjects on *DSM III-R* criteria for dementia and on NINCDS-ADRDA criteria for AD. These subjects were followed for at least 10 years, and the study included three waves from 1993 through 1998. The study generated a global incidence rate for MCI of 9.9 per 1000 person years. Mild cognitive impairment predicted AD with an annual rate of 8.3%; however, it was quite unstable across time, and approximately 40% of the MCI group reverted to normal. They concluded that MCI is a useful concept because of its ability to predict AD in a rather specific fashion, but they believe that it can be unstable, particularly when the diagnosis is based on psychometric tests which themselves can be unstable. This study was particularly well done and, once again, emphasized the importance of the clinical characterization of subjects in addition to the use of neuropsychological testing.

PREDICTORS OF PROGRESSION

While subjects must have a memory impairment to be classified as having MCI, certain factors have been identified which predict a more rapid progression to dementia and AD. The Mayo group reported that apolipoprotein E $\varepsilon 4$ (*APOE-4*) carriers were more likely to progress to AD than were noncarriers (Petersen et al., 1995). Tierney and colleagues (1996) found that *APOE-4* also predicted progression, but only when used in conjunction with performance on a memory test, and the latter actually proved to be more useful. The *APOE* finding has been somewhat variable and likely is only a weak predictor of clinical progression.

Predictors of progression for individuals in the Washington University studies included the collateral source–derived history of compromised function in everyday activities compared with former abilities, and the poor performance of the individual on most psychometric measures, especially those tapping episodic memory (e.g., paragraph recall) (Morris et al., 2001). Bowen and colleagues (1997) in Seattle did not find neuropsychological tests to be useful as a predictor of progression. The NYU group has summarized several years of their longitudinal studies and concluded that a small set of neuropsychological tests, especially a paragraph delayed recall test, predicted decliners from nondecliners after accounting for age, sex, education, follow-up interval, and global clinical status (Flicker et al., 1991; Kluger et al., 1999).

Collie and Maruff (2000) from Australia argue for the importance of assessing a memory decline rather than a single cross-sectional measure of memory impairment. They evaluated word list delayed-recall five times over a 2-year period and identified 35 subjects with declining scores and 66 with nondeclining scores. They argued for the value of a memory change over time as being particularly important and indicated that this measure would avoid the possibility of misclassifying elderly subjects based on a single cognitive assessment (Collie and Maruff, 2000). While this is an important issue, the follow-up interval in this study was too short to justify this conclusion since the clinical outcome of these subjects is not known. Nevertheless, the concept of longitudinal memory assessment has merit.

Devanand and colleagues (2000) from Columbia found that subjects with low olfaction scores who reported no subjective problems with smelling were more likely to develop AD than were other patients. They argued that since olfaction is represented in medial temporal lobe structures in the brain likely to be involved in early AD, olfaction may be a useful clinical measure to evaluate and follow subjects at risk.

Neuroimaging has become a major focus of research in incipient AD. Neuroimaging studies can measure either structural or functional parameters (see Chapters 6 and 7). The greatest amount of work has been done on the basis of structural neuroimaging (DeCarli et al., 1990; Jack et al., 1997; Kaye et al., 1997; Fox et al., 1998). Studies have indicated that MRI-based volumetric measurements of the hippocampus can differentiate normal subjects from those with MCI and AD (Jack et al., 1999). Measurements of the entorhinal cortex also have been proposed (Killiany et al., 2000; Xu et al., 2000). Investigators feel that since the entorhinal cortex is the site of earliest pathology in AD, this structure should manifest the earliest volumetric changes in incipient AD (Killiany et al., 2000). Some studies have indicated that the volume of the entorhinal cortex is a useful predictor of progression from MCI to AD, while others have argued that measurements of the entorhinal cortex are no better than hippocampal measures (Xu et al., 2000) (see Chapter 6). Part of this argument revolves around the precision by which these two regions can be accurately measured.

Jack and colleagues (2000) have evaluated hippocampal formation and have shown that the rate of change mirrors progression in clinical states. Whole brain atrophy has also been proposed as a useful measure of clinical progression (Fox et al., 1999, 2001). Fox and colleagues have developed an exquisite technique for measuring changes in whole brain volume using a technique called "boundary shift integral" (Fox et al., 2001). This technique uses a very precise measure of voxel by voxel registration to assess volumetric changes over time. This measurement technique is currently being applied to MCI subjects.

Several of the currently ongoing treatment trials for MCI are using quantitative imaging as a marker of disease progression. Since serial data are available on hippocampal and whole brain changes in normal, MCI, and AD subjects, these measures may be useful as markers of disease progression.

Functional neuroimaging has also been applied to the assessment of early AD (Small et al., 1995; Reiman et al., 1996). Johnson and colleagues (1998; Johnson and Albert, 2000) at Harvard have used single photon emission computed tomography (SPECT) measurements to predict progression and have demonstrated usefulness in detecting early AD-like patterns of hypoperfusion (see Chapter 7). Small et al. (1995) and Reiman et al. (1996) have demonstrated positron emission tomography (PET) abnormalities in metabolism in presymptomatic family members of subjects with AD who are *APOE-4* carriers. While these data do not apply directly to MCI, since the subjects are functioning normally, they suggest that these patterns may be useful in MCI as well.

Finally, Kantarci et al. (2000) have demonstrated MR spectroscopy (MRS) changes in myoinositol/creatine ratios in MCI. The myoinositol/creatine ratio was increased in MCI relative to normal control subjects and further elevated in AD relative to MCI. The *N*-acetyl aspartate/creatine ratio declined only in AD relative to MCI. Presumably *N*-acetyl aspartate represents noronal integrity, and myoinositol may reflect glial activity.

It is likely that a combination of clinical, genetic, and neuroimaging markers may combine to be particularly useful in predicting which subjects with MCI are destined to progress to AD.

Perhaps therapeutic strategies can be tailored to certain progression patterns in subjects allowing for more effective treatments in carefully selected subjects.

SUMMARY

Mild cognitive impairment as currently conceived by most investigators is a clinical entity that represents a transitional state between the cognitive changes of normal aging and the earliest presentations of clinically probable AD as depicted by published criteria. Controversy exists as to how MCI can best be defined. At present, most longitudinal studies, especially the clinical trials currently under way, use a variation of the criteria discussed in this chapter. The difficulties result from the operationalization of these criteria. For example, the issue of a memory complaint concerns the subject's awareness of a memory problem and the importance of corroboration of this concern by an informant. Therefore, any hint of a memory problem should be pursued. This does not mean that every person with a suggestion of a memory problem has MCI, but clinicians should have a low threshold for pursuing these evaluations.

The objective memory impairment that is part of the criteria is determined by a combination of the history from the subject and an informant, supplemented with neuropsychological testing. The degree of impairment is assessed neuropsychologically, but the result of the impairment is determined by the clinician through the exam and interview. Consequently, no single cutoff score determines the memory impairment. Rather, the degree of impairment is gauged relative to appropriate normative data, and the importance of this degree of impairment is assessed clinically. In a similar vein, the largely normal indices of general cognitive function and activities of daily living are determined by the clinical history and exam and are complemented by neuropsychological testing and activities of daily living scales. Performance on these measures may be statistically lower for MCI subjects than for normal control subjects, but the clinical impact of these neuropsychological findings is of insufficient magnitude to convince the clinician that the person is demented. Since most definitions of dementia require cognitive impairment in memory and non-memory domains with a resulting functional impact, clinicians evaluating MCI subjects do not believe that this criterion is met. This can be a contentious issue in the literature.

Finally, and most important, the clinician does not feel that the person with the amnestic form of MCI meets the criteria for dementia. Therefore, most clinicians are not comfortable in diagnosing probable AD. This may change as the threshold for dementia diagnosis increasingly evolves to incorporate earlier stages of the illness. In addition, the evolution of sensitive detection methods (e.g., measures of episodic memory, combined with collateral source-based assessments) or, ultimately, a surrogate marker for AD, will improve confidence in the early diagnosis of AD.

When the criteria for MCI are discussed from this perspective, the diagnostic process is quite similar to that used in making the diagnosis of dementia by *DSM III-R* or *DSM IV* or the diagnosis of probable AD by NINCDS-ADRDA criteria. These criteria do not incorporate cutoff scores on neuropsychological tests or activities of daily living scales; rather, they involve the judgment of the clinician. In a similar fashion, the MCI criteria proposed here outline specific aspects of the clinical presentation of the subject in this prodromal stage without specifying particular tests, instruments, or cutoff scores. The criteria are designed to emphasize the early cognitive presentation of either an incipient dementia or AD.

The ultimate importance of the concept of MCI may not reside in the specific operationalization of the criteria. There are likely to be legitimate variations on these criteria as a function of the clinical setting and the subject population. The ultimate result of the study of the clinical disorder such as MCI may be derived from its ability to draw the clinician's attention to the earliest presentation of a cognitive impairment. As the field of aging and dementia moves forward, these subjects will become candidates for treatment interventions designed to slow or halt the underlying progression of the pathologic process.

References

Bassett, S.S., and M.F. Folstein. (1993). Memory complaint, memory performance and psychiatric diagnosis: a community study. *J Geriatr Psychiatry Neurol* 6:105–111.

Berg, L., D.W. McKeel Jr., J.P. Miller, M. Storandt, E.H. Rubin, J.C. Morris, J. Baty, M. Coats, J. Norton, A.M. Goate, J.L. Price, M. Gearing, S.S. Mirra, and A.M. Saunders. (1998). Clinicopathologic studies in cognitively healthy aging and Alzheimer disease: relation of histologic markers to dementia severity, age, sex, and apolipoprotein E genotype. *Arch Neurol* 55:326–335.

Bowen, J., L. Teri, W. Kukull, W. McCormick, S.M. McCurry, and E.B. Larson. (1997). Progression to dementia in patients with isolated memory loss. *Lancet* 349(9054):763–765.

Bozoki, A., B. Giordani, J.L. Heidebrink, S. Berent, and N.L. Foster. (2001). Mild cognitive impairments predict dementia in nondemented elderly patients with memory loss. *Arch Neurol* 58:411–416.

Carr, D.B., S. Gray, J. Baty, and J.C. Morris. (2000). The value of informant vs. individual's complaints of memory impairment in early dementia. *Neurology* 55:1724–1726.

Collie, A., and P. Maruff. (2000). The neuropsychology of preclinical Alzheimer's disease and mild cognitive impairment. *Neurosci Biobehav Rev* 24(3):365–374.

Crook, T., R.T. Bartus, S.H. Ferris, P. Whitehouse, G.D. Cohen, and S. Gershon. (1986). Age-associated memory impairment: proposed diagnostic criteria and measures of clinical change—report of a National Institute of Mental Health Work Group. *Devel Neuropsychol* 2:261–276.

Daly, E., D. Zaitchik, M. Copeland, J. Schmahmann, J. Gunther, and M. Albert. (2000). Predicting conversion to Alzheimer disease using standardized clinical information. *Arch Neurol* 57(5):675–680.

Dartigues, J.F., C. Fabrigoule, L. Letenneur, H. Amieva, F. Thiessard, and J.M. Orgogozo. (1997). Epidemiologie des troubles de la memoire. *Therapie* 52:503–506.

DeCarli, C., J.A. Kaye, B. Horwitz, and S.I. Rapoport. (1990). Critical analysis of the use of computer-assisted transverse axial tomography to study human brain in aging and dementia of the alzheimer type. *Neurology* 40:872–883.

Devanand, D.P., M. Folz, M. Gorlyn, J.R. Moeller, and Y. Stern. (1997). Questionable dementia: clinical course and predictors of outcome. *J Am Geriatr Soc* 45:321–328.

Devanand, D.P., K.S. Michaels-Marston, X. Liu, G.H. Pelton, M. Padilla, K. Marder, K. Bell, Y. Stern, and R. Mayeux. (2000). Olfactory deficits in patients with mild cognitive impairment predict Alzheimer's disease at follow-up. *Am J Psychiatry* 157(9):1399–1405.

Diagnostic and Statistical Manual of Mental Disorders, 4th ed. (1994). Washington, DC: American Psychiatric Association. [*DSM- IV*]

Flicker, C., S.H. Ferris, and B. Reisberg. (1991). Mild cognitive impairment in the elderly: predictors of dementia. *Neurology* 41:1006–1009.

Folstein, M.F., S.E. Folstein, and P.R. McHugh. (1975). "Mini-Mental State." A practical method for grading the cognitive state of patients for the clinician. *J Psychiatr Res* 12(3):189–198.

Fox, N.C., E.K. Warrington, A.L. Seiffer, S.K. Agnew, and M.N. Rossor. (1998). Presymptomatic cognitive deficits in individuals at risk of familial Alzheimer's disease: a longitudinal prospective study. *Brain* 121(Pt 9):1631–1639.

Fox, N.C., R.I. Scahill, W.R. Crum, and M.N. Rossor. (1999). Correlation between rates of brain atrophy and cognitive decline in AD. *Neurology* 52:1687–1689.

Fox, N.C., W.R. Crum, R.I. Scahill, J.M. Stevens, J.C. Janssen, and M.N. Rossor. (2001). Imaging of onset and progression of Alzheimer's disease with voxel-compression mapping of serial magnetic resonance images. *Lancet* 358:201–205.

Geerlings, M.I., C. Jonker, L.M. Bouter, H.J. Ader, and B. Schmand. (1999). Association between memory complaints and incident Alzheimer's disease in elderly people with normal baseline cognition. *Am J Psychiatr* 156:531–537.

Goldman, W.P., and J.C. Morris. (2001). Evidence that age-associated memory impairment is not a normal variant of aging. *Alzheimer Dis Assoc Disord* 15(2):72–79.

Graham, J.E., K. Rockwood, B.L. Beattie, R. Eastwood, S. Gauthier, H. Tuokko, and I. McDowell. (1997). Prevalence and severity of cognitive impairment with and without dementia in an elderly population. *Lancet* 349:1793–1796.

Ivnik, R.J., J.F. Malec, G.E. Smith, E.G. Tangalos, R.C. Petersen, E. Kokmen, and L.T. Kurland. (1992). Mayo's Older Americans Normative Studies: WAIS-R, WMS-R and AVLT norms for ages 56 through 97. *Clin Neuropsychol* 6(Suppl):1–104.

Ivnik, R.J., G.E. Smith, J.F. Malec, R.C. Petersen, E. Kokmen, and E.G. Tangalos. (1994). Mayo Cognitive Factor Scales: distinguishing normal and clinical samples by profile variability. *Neuropsychology* 8(2):203–209.

Ivnik, R.J., G.E. Smith, J.F. Malec, R.C. Petersen, and E.G. Tangalos. (1995). Long-term stability and intercorrelations of cognitive abilities in older persons. *Psychol Assess* 7(2):155–161.

Ivnik, R.J., G.E. Smith, J.A. Lucas, R.C. Petersen, B.F. Boeve, E. Kokmen, and E.G. Tangalos. (1999). Testing normal older people three or four times at 1- to 2-year intervals: defining normal variance. *Neuropsychology* 13(1):121–127.

Jack, C.R. Jr., R.C. Petersen, Y.C. Xu, S.C. Waring, P.C. O'Brien, E.C. Tangalos, G.E. Smith, R.J. Ivnik, and E. Kokmen. (1997). Medial temporal atrophy on MRI in normal aging and very mild Alzheimer's disease. *Neurology* 49(3):786–794.

Jack, C.R. Jr., R.C. Petersen, Y.C. Xu, P.C. O'Brien, G.E. Smith, R.J. Ivnik, B.F. Boeve, S.C. Waring, E.G. Tangalos, and E. Kokmen. (1999). Prediction of AD with MRI-based hippocampal volume in mild cognitive impairment. *Neurology* 52(7):1397–1403.

Jack, C.R. Jr., R.C. Petersen, Y. Xu, P.C. O'Brien, G.E. Smith, R.J. Ivnik, B.F. Boeve, E.G. Tangalos, and E. Kokmen. (2000). Rates of hippocampal atrophy correlate with change in clinical status in aging and AD. *Neurology* 55(4):484–489.

Johnson, K.A., and M.S. Albert. (2000). Perfusion abnormalities in prodromal AD. *Neurobiol Aging* 21:289–292.

Johnson, K.A., K.J. Jones, J.A. Becker, A. Satlin, B.L. Holman, and M.S. Albert. (1998). Preclinical prediction of Alzheimer's disease using SPECT. *Neurology* 50:1563–1571.

Kantarci, K., C.R. Jack Jr., Y.C. Xu, N.G. Campeau, P.C. O'Brien, G.E. Smith, R.J. Ivnik, B.F. Boeve, E. Kokmen, E.G. Tangalos, and R.C. Petersen. (2000). Regional metabolic patterns in mild cognitive impairment and Alzheimer's disease: a 1H MRS study. *Neurology* 55(2):210–217.

Kaye, J.A., T. Swihart, D. Howieson, A. Dame, M.M. Moore, T. Karnos, R. Camicioli, M. Ball, B. Oken, and G. Sexton. (1997). Volume loss of the hippocampus and temporal lobe in healthy elderly persons destined to develop dementia. *Neurology* 48:1297–1304.

Killiany, R.J., T. Gomez-Isla, M. Moss, R. Kikinis, T. Sandor, F. Jolesz, R. Tanzi, K. Jones, B.T. Hyman, and M.S. Albert. (2000). Use of structural magnetic resonance imaging to predict who will get Alzheimer's disease. *Ann Neurol* 47.430–439.

Kluger, A., S.H. Ferris, J. Golomb, M.S. Mittelman, and B. Reisberg. (1999). Neuropsychological prediction of decline to dementia in nondemented elderly. *J Geriatr Psychiatry Neurol* 12:168–179.

Kral, V.A. (1962). Senescent forgetfulness: benign and malignant. *Can Med Assoc J* 86:257–260.

Larrieu, S., L. Letenneur, J.M. Orgogozo, C. Fabrigoule, H. Amieva, N. Le Carret, P. Barberger-Gateau, and J.F. Dartigues. (In press). Incidence and outcome of mild cognitive impairment in a population-based prospective cohort.

Levy, R. (1994). Aging-associated cognitive decline. *Int Psychogeriatr* 6:63–68.

McKhann, G., D. Drachman, M. Folstein, R. Katzman, D. Price, and E.M. Stadlan. (1984). Clinical diagnosis of Alzheimer's disease: report of the NINCDS-ADRDA work group under the auspices of Department of Health and Human Services Task Force on Alzheimer's Disease. *Neurology* 34:939–944.

Morris, J.C. (1993). The Clinical Dementia Rating (CDR): Current version and scoring rules. *Neurology* 43:2412–2414.

Morris, J.C., S. Edland, C. Clark, D. Galasko, E. Koss, R. Mohs, G. van Belle, G. Fillenbaum, and A. Heyman. (1993). The consortium to establish a registry for Alzheimer's disease (CERAD). Part IV: Rates of cognitive change in the longitudinal assessment of probable Alzheimer's disease. *Neurology* 43:2457–2465.

Morris, J.C., M. Storandt, D.W. McKeel Jr., E.H. Rubin, J.L. Price, E.A. Grant, and L. Berg. (1996). Cerebral amyloid deposition and diffuse plaques in "normal" aging: evidence for presymptomatic and very mild Alzheimer's disease. *Neurology* 46:707–719.

Morris, J.C., M. Storandt, J.P. Miller, D.W. McKeel, J.L. Price, E.H. Rubin, and L. Berg. (2001). Mild cognitive impairment represents early-stage Alzheimer's disease. *Arch Neurol* 58:397–405.

O'Brien, J.T., B. Beats, K. Hill, R. Howard, B. Sahakian, and R. Levy. (1992). Do subjective memory complaints precede dementia? A three-year follow-up of patients with supposed "benign senescent forgetfulness." *Int J Geriatr Psychiatry* 7:481–486.

Petersen, R.C. (1995). Normal aging, mild cognitive impairment, and early Alzheimer's disease. *Neurologist* 1:326–344.

Petersen, R.C. (2000a). Mild cognitive impairment: transition between aging and Alzheimer's disease. *Neurologia* 15:93–101.

Petersen, R.C. (2000b). Mild cognitive impairment or questionable dementia? [editorial; comment]. *Arch Neurol* 57:643–644.

Petersen, R.C., R. Doody, A. Kurz, R. Mohs, J.C. Morris, P.V. Rabins, K.
Ritchie, M. Russor, L. Thal, and B. Winblad. (2001). Current concepts
in mild cognitive impairment. *Arch Neurol* 58:1985–1992.

Petersen, R.C., E. Kokmen, E. Tangalos, R.J. Ivnik, and L.T. Kurland.
(1990). Mayo Clinic Alzheimer's Disease Patient Registry. *Aging* 2:408–
415.

Petersen, R.C., G.E. Smith, R.J. Ivnik, E.G. Tangalos, D.J. Schaid, S.N. Thibodeau, E. Kokmen, S.C. Waring, and L.T. Kurland. (1995). Apolipoprotein E status as a predictor of the development of Alzheimer's disease in memory-impaired individuals. *JAMA* 273:1274–1278.

Petersen, R.C., G.E. Smith, S.C. Waring, R.J. Ivnik, E.G. Tangalos, and E.
Kokmen. (1999). Mild cognitive impairment: clinical characterization
and outcome. *Arch Neurol* 56:303–308.

Reiman, E.M., R.J. Caselli, L.S. Yun, K. Chen, D. Bandy, S. Minoshima, S.N.
Thibodeau, and D. Osborne. (1996). Preclinical evidence of Alzheimer's disease in persons homozygous for the *E4* allele for apolipoprotein E. *N Engl J Med* 334(12):752–758.

Reisberg, B., S.H. Ferris, M.J. de Leon, and T. Crook. (1982). The Global
Deterioration Scale for assessment of primary degenerative dementia.
Am J Psychiatry 139:1136–1139.

Rey, A. (1964). L'examen clinique en psychologie. Paris: Presses Universitaires de France.

Riedel-Heller, S.G., H. Matschinger, A. Schork, and M.C. Angermeyer.
(1999). Do memory complaints indicate the presence of cognitive impairment? Results of a field study. *Eur Arch Psychiatry Clin Neurosci* 249:
197–204.

Ritchie, K., D. Leibovici, B. Ledesert, and J. Touchon. (1996). A typology
of sub-clinical senescent cognitive disorder. *Br J Psychiatry* 168(4):470–
476.

Ritchie, K., S. Artero, and J. Touchon. (2000). Classification criteria for
mild cognitive impairment: a population-based validation study. *Neurology* 56:37–42.

Rubin, E.H., M. Storandt, P. Miller, D.A. Kinscherf, E.A. Grant, J.C. Morris,
and L. Berg. (1998). A prospective study of cognitive function and
onset of dementia in cognitively healthy elders. *Arch Neurol* 55:395–401.

Schmand, B., C. Jonker, C. Hooijr, and J. Lindeboom. (1996). Subjective
memory complaints may announce dementia. *Neurology* 46:121–125.

Schofield, P.W., D. Jacobs, K. Marder, M. Sanon, and Y. Stern. (1997a). The
validity of new memory complaints in the elderly. *Arch Neurol* 54:756–
759.

Schofield, P.W., K. Marder, G. Dooneief, D.M. Jacobs, M. Sano, and Y. Stern.
(1997b). Association of subjective memory complaints with subsequent
cognitive decline in community-dwelling elderly individuals with baseline cognitive impairment. *Am J Psychiatr* 154:609–615.

Small, G.W., J.C. Mazziotta, M.T. Collins, L.R. Baxter, M.E. Phelps, M.A.
Mandelkern, A. Kaplan, A. La Rue, C.F. Adamson, L. Chang, B.H.
Guze, E.H. Corder, A.M. Saunders, J.L. Haines, M.A. Pericak-Vance,
and A.D. Roses. (1995). Apolipoprotein E type 4 allele and cerebral

glucose metabolism in relatives at risk for familial Alzheimer disease. *JAMA* 273(12):942–947.

Smith, G., R.J. Ivnik, R.C. Petersen, J.F. Malec, E. Kokmen, and E. Tangalos. (1991). Age-associated memory impairment diagnoses: problems of reliability and concerns for terminology. *Psychol Aging* 6(4):551–558.

Smith, G.E., R.J. Ivnik, J.F. Malec, E. Kokmen, E.G. Tangalos, and L.T. Kurland. (1992). Mayo's Older Americans Normative Studies (MOANS): factor structure of a core battery. *Psychol Assess* 4(3):382–390.

Smith, G.E., R.J. Ivnik, J.F. Malec, E. Kokmen, E. Tangalos, R.C. Petersen, and E. Atkinson. (1994a). Psychometric properties of the Mattis Dementia Rating Scale. *Assessment* 1(2):115–123.

Smith, G.E., R.J. Ivnik, J.F. Malec, R.C. Petersen, E. Kokmen, and E.G. Tangalos. (1994b). Mayo cognitive factors scales: derivation of a short battery and norms for factor scores. *Neuropsychology* 8(2):194–202.

Smith, G.E., R.C. Petersen, R.J. Ivnik, J.F. Malec, and E.G. Tangalos. (1996). Subjective memory complaints, psychological distress, and longitudinal change in objective memory performance. *Psychol Aging* 11(2):272–279.

Smith, G.E., D.L. Bohac, R.J. Ivnik, and J.F. Malec. (1997). Using word recognition tests to estimate premorbid IQ in early dementia: longitudinal data. *J International Neuropsychol Soc* 3(6):528–533.

Smith, G.E., E. Kokmen, and P.C. O'Brien. (2000). Risk factors for nursing home placement in a population-based dementia cohort. *J Am Geriatr Soc* 48(5):519–525.

Tierney, M.C., J.P. Szalai, W.G. Snow, and R.H. Fisher. (1996). The prediction of Alzheimer disease: the role of patient and informant perceptions of cognitive deficits. *Arch Neurol* 53:423–427.

Tierney, M.C., J.P. Szalai, W.G. Snow, R.H. Fisher, A. Nores, G. Nadon, E. Dunn, and P.H. St. George-Hyslop. (1996a). Prediction of probable Alzheimer's disease in memory-impaired patients: a prospective longitudinal study. *Neurology* 46(3):661–665.

Tierney, M.C., J.P. Szalai, W.G. Snow, R.H. Fisher, T. Tsuda, H. Chi, D.R. McLachlan, and P.H. St. George-Hyslop. (1996b). A prospective study of the clinical utility of ApoE genotype in the prediction of outcome in patients with memory impairment. *Neurology* 46(1):149–154.

Tobiansky, R., R. Blizard, G. Livingston, and A. Mann. (1995). The Gospel Oak Study stage IV: the clinical relevance of subjective memory impairment in older people. *Psychol Med* 25:779–786.

Wechsler, D.A. (1987). Wechsler Memory Scale–Revised. New York: Psychological Corporation.

Weintraub, S. (1986). The Record of Independent Living: an informant-completed measure of activities of daily living and behavior in elderly patients with cognitive impairment. *Am J Alzheimer's Care Related Disord* 7:35–39.

Xu, Y., C.R. Jack Jr., P.C. O'Brien, E. Kokmen, G.E. Smith, R.J. Ivnik, B.F. Boeve, E.G. Tangalos, and R.C. Petersen. (2000). Usefulness of MRI measures of entorhinal cortex versus hippocampus in AD. *Neurology* 54(9):1760–1767.

CHAPTER 3

Neuropsychiatric Symptoms

JEFFREY L. CUMMINGS

It is increasingly imperative that Alzheimer's disease (AD) be detected as early in its clinical course as possible. The goals of treatment of AD are to slow the progress and control the symptoms, thus increasing the period of relatively preserved function while decreasing the period of disability. Treatments are most likely to be successful if they are begun while patients are in the mildest phase of the disease. Antioxidants, (such as vitamin E and selegiline), nonsteroidal anti-inflammatory drugs (NSAIDs), and estrogen all appear to slow the progress of AD and may improve existing symptoms. Likewise, cholinesterase inhibitors and cholinergic agonists may improve cognitive and behavioral symptoms, or they may temporarily slow the rate of cognitive decline. Current laboratory efforts to discover agents that will reduce the production of amyloid, increase the excretion of amyloid, reduce the aggregation of amyloid, or enhance neuronal survival all promise to slow the progress of AD. This emerging armamentarium will be of greatest benefit if patients can be detected and treated early in the course of the disease.

A variety of approaches have been developed to identify patients who are at risk for AD or who are in the earliest phases of the illness. Risk factors include age, female gender, apolipoprotein E-4 (*APOE-4*) genotype, history of head injury, low educational level, limited intelligence, small head size, and lack of estrogen replacement therapy in postmenopausal women (Cummings et al., 1998). Early detection has emphasized loss of memory, particularly semantic memory, plus disturbances in other effort-demanding tasks, such as copying complex constructions, confrontation naming, verbal fluency, set shifting, and verbal abstraction (Parks and Zek, 1993).

Neuroimaging changes also have been sought as early markers of AD. Temporal lobe atrophy (Jobst et al., 1992a), increased ventricular volume and sylvian sulcal enlargement (Förstl et al., 1995), reduced glucose metabolism in the parietal association cortex (Haxby et al., 1986), and reduced blood flow in the posterior parietotemporal cortex in combination with temporal atrophy (Jobst et al., 1992b) have been promoted as alterations occurring early in the course of AD. Changes in complex, everyday behaviors also have been emphasized as possible early manifestations of AD (Agency for Health Care Policy and Research, 1996).

Relatively few studies have investigated the possible role of neuropsychiatric symptoms or changes in mood, personality, and emotion as potential early markers of the presence of AD. This chapter reviews the evidence suggesting that these changes may be markers of the onset of AD. First, the difference between risk factors and early events of the illness is considered. Next, the relationship of late-onset depression and depression with cognitive changes to AD is examined. The interaction between behavior and genotype is described. Then, the occurrence of depressive and nondepressive behavioral alterations early in the course of AD is presented. The pathobiology of AD and its relevance to the early occurrence of emotional alterations are discussed. Finally, the assessment of behavioral changes in AD and the role of neuropsychiatric symptoms in future research in AD are considered.

RISK FACTORS VERSUS HARBINGER BEHAVIORAL CHANGES

Several case-control studies have found depression to be a risk factor for AD (French et al., 1985; Shalat et al., 1987; Broe et al., 1990; Kokmen et al., 1991). The methodology of these studies, however, makes it difficult to determine whether depression was more common among the AD member of matched cases because it occurred as a harbinger event immediately before the onset of AD or because it represented a risk factor that increased the vulnerability of the patient to the later occurrence of AD. Broe and colleagues (1990) found that depression occurring within the last 10 years was a risk factor for AD, whereas depression occurring more than 10 years before the onset of AD was not. This suggests that depression may be an early or preclinical event in the course of AD. Devanand et al. (1996) found that the presence of depression increased the likelihood of the emergence of dementia (primarily AD) in an elderly population over the next two and one-half years by approximately threefold. Liston (1977) retrospectively examined the medical records of 50 patients with the diagnosis of presenile dementia (predominantly AD) and noted that half had symptoms of major depressive disorder before their diagnosis, and one-fourth had depressive spectrum diagnoses. Jost and Grossberg (1996) found that depressive symptoms were evident in 50% of patients approximately 2 years before the diagnosis of AD. Baker et al. (1991), reported that 31% of patients with AD had a preceding diagnosis of depression, and Agbayewa (1986) found depression in the past histories of 78% of AD patients. While it is possible that the occurrence of depression is a marker for neuronal dysfunction, cerebral vascular disease, or other condition that increases the patient's risk of manifesting AD, the evidence is also consistent with depression as an initial event heralding the imminent development of AD.

Two studies suggest that personality changes might also be regarded, like depression, as harbinger events. These emerged in case-control studies and are subject to the same ambiguities of interpretation as noted for depressive disorders. Broe and colleagues (1990) found that physical underactivity in both the past 10 years and as a lifetime characteristic was more common among AD patients than among matched controls. The relationship was stronger for the 10-year period before the onset of AD. Kokmen et al. (1991) reported that a diagnosis of personality disorder was more common among AD patients than among controls. Personality disorders were not further defined but could include features of "organic personality disorder" associated with neurological illness.

Thus, case-control studies of risk factors for AD raise a challenging issue with regard to data interpretation. The behavioral changes noted—depression and personality alterations—may be manifestations of cerebral changes that increase vulnerability to AD, or they may be harbinger events that emerge as risk factors because they preceded the identification of cognitive changes. Longitudinal studies of elderly patients with late-onset depressive disorders or personality changes may provide further insight into this issue.

DEMENTIA OF DEPRESSION AND ALZHEIMER'S DISEASE

The concept of "pseudodementia" embraces at least two clinically distinguishable subgroups. In the first, the patients complain of cognitive impairment, give frequent "I don't know" answers in response to mental status tests, perform at higher-than-expected levels in activities of daily living, and can sometimes be shown to have normal performances on cognitive tests when their cooperation can be obtained. The second syndrome, also known as the dementia of depression (DOD), is characterized by failures on cognitive tests despite satisfactory effort, impairments on both bedside assessments of mental status and neuropsychological tests, and broad-ranging abnormalities of mental state, including disturbances of memory, abstract reasoning, attention, and perception (McHugh and Folstein, 1979; Wells, 1979; Caine, 1981; Cummings, 1989).

There is a reasonable consensus in the literature suggesting that the first type of pseudodementia recovers with treatment and is unlikely to mark the occurrence of a dementing illness. Controversy, however, surrounds the fate of the individual with DOD. Two longitudinal studies that followed patients with DOD for a 2-year period found no increased prevalence of dementia among patients with DOD, compared to depressed patients without coexistent cognitive impairment (Rabins et al., 1984; La Rue et al., 1986). Similarly, Sachdev and colleagues (1990) completed a longitudinal follow-up of a group of 19 patients with assorted psychiatric illnesses and concomitant cognitive compromise. Of the 19, a total of 8 had major depression at the time of initial assessment, 5 had bipolar illness, and 6 had schizophrenia. At the time of reexamination—from 2 to 14 years after initial assessment—only one patient had developed a dementia syndrome. This patient was diagnosed initially as suffering from schizophrenia and progressed to develop Huntington's disease. One patient with an initial diagnosis of major depression continued to be depressed and had possible dementia at the time of his death 2 years after initial assessment.

In contrast, Kral and Emery (1989) reported a follow-up study of 44 elderly patients with DOD whom they had followed for 4 to 18 years (average of 8 years). At the time of the follow-up observation, 39 of the 44 (89%) had developed AD.

Two other studies bear on this important issue. Pearlson and colleagues (1989) assessed the cognitive deficits and cerebral atrophy as measured on computerized tomograms of a group of patients with DOD and a matched group with depression unaccompanied by cognitive impairment. The two groups were compared to a group of patients with established AD and a group of normal elderly controls. Patients with DOD clustered near AD patients in both their measures of cerebral atrophy and their patterns of cognitive deficits. Of 11 patients reexamined after a 2-year interval, 1 developed a dementing disorder. In a recent study, Alexopoulos and colleagues (1993) followed a group of 57 elderly patients hospitalized for major depression: 27 with DOD and 30 with depression unaccompanied by a dementia syndrome. Patients were followed for an average of nearly 3 years, and during that period, 43% of DOD patients developed an irreversible dementing disorder, whereas 12% of patients with an initial diagnosis of major depression without dementia became demented. Of the 10 subjects who developed dementia during the follow-up period, 6 had AD, 2 had vascular dementia, and 2 had dementia syndromes of undetermined etiology.

Differences among studies in terminology and clinical diagnosis of both AD and depression make it difficult to draw firm conclusions from the existing literature on DOD regarding the frequency of ensuing dementia, but, at a minimum, it suggests a heterogeneous outcome of DOD with some patients progressing to a dementia syndrome. Research in this area will need to distinguish between early-onset and late-onset depressions; recognize the phenomenologic heterogeneity among late-life depressions; and seek neuropsychiatric, neuropsychologic, and biological markers of patients who experience DOD as precursory to the evolution of AD. The importance of identifying a group of DOD patients whose latent AD is made manifest by the occurrence of the depression syndrome is obvious since preventive therapies or drugs that slow the progression of AD could be administered to these patients with delay of onset of the dementia.

NONDEPRESSIVE NEUROPSYCHIATRIC SYMPTOMS PRECEDING ONSET OF ALZHEIMER'S DISEASE

Agbayewa (1986) found higher rates of paranoid disorders (17.5%) in the past histories of patients with AD than in normal controls. Similarly, Lesser and colleagues (1989) assessed 40 patients who had their first psychotic episode when they were older than age 45. All patients were nondemented at the time of study onset. Three of the 40 patients developed dementia within a short period of time, suggesting that the psychosis was the initial manifestation of the dementia. Two of the patients developed frontotemporal degeneration, and one manifested AD. In a study by Jost and Grossberg (1996), 20% of patients had paranoid ideation approximately 15 months before the diagnosis of AD was established. Crystal and colleagues (1988) described a 70-year-old woman who developed AD within 1 year of the onset of formed visual hallucinations. Baker and colleagues (1991) found that 14.6% of patients had a history of preceding anxiety disorder (usually late-onset) preceding the onset of their AD. These studies suggest that late-onset behavioral changes of a variety of types may precede the onset of AD.

EARLY NEUROPSYCHIATRIC SYMPTOMS AND *APOE* GENOTYPE

The *APOE-4* genotype is a risk factor for sporadic and familial AD (Corder et al., 1993). The type 4 apolipoprotein may exert its effect through enhancement of aggregation of amyloid in the brain: Apolipoprotein is present in neuritic plaques, and amyloid peptide deposition is more severe in patients with this genotype (Cummings et al., 1998). The presence of the *APOE-4* genotype in patients with late-onset neuropsychiatric disorders may help identify those who are in the prodromal or preliminary phases of AD. Zubenko and colleagues (1996) reported that depressed patients with psychotic features had a frequency of the *e-4* apolipoprotein allele nearly four times greater than had depressed patients without psychotic features. Patients with the *e-4* allele did not have more severe cognitive impairment during their depressive episodes than patients without the *e-4* allele. Krishnan and coworkers (1996) also found a higher frequency of the *e-4* allele among patients with late-onset depression, suggesting that some were at high risk for AD. Those with the *e-4* allele also had lower Mini-Mental State Examination (MMSE) scores (Folstein et al., 1975) than did those without, further supporting the idea that some of the patients were likely to develop AD. Heidrich and colleagues (1997), however, found no increase of the *APOE-4* genotype in late-onset over that in early-onset depression. Steffens and coworkers (1997) confirmed the increased rates of depression before diagnosis of AD and increased rates of *APOE-4* genotypes among AD patients; they did not find an interaction between depression and genotype, suggesting that the two factors were independent risk factors.

These data are inconclusive in determining the relationship between *APOE-4* genotype, depression, and AD. Individuals with late-onset depression and an *e-4* allele are at increased risk for AD; the degree to which these patients are overrepresented among patients with late-onset depressions requires clarification.

DEPRESSION AND ANXIETY AS MANIFESTATIONS OF EARLY ALZHEIMER'S DISEASE

The DOD, as noted, precede the onset of AD. However, in DOD there is an interval of normal, cognitive function and euthymia between the DOD episode and the emergence of AD. In this section, the occurrence of depression in concert with mild cognitive impairment in the first phase of AD is examined.

Among a group of 50 patients with mild dementia (primarily AD) and 134 normal elderly control subjects, Wands and co-workers (1990) reported probable or possible depression in 28% of patients and 3% of controls; 38% of dementia patients and 9% of controls had a probable or possible diagnosis of an anxiety disorder. In patients with global deterioration scores of 3, corresponding to mild dementia, Reisberg and colleagues (1989) reported that 21.4% of patients exhibited depressed mood, making statements, such as "I wish I were dead." Assessing anxiety symptoms, the authors found that 42.9% of patients had anxiety about upcoming events, while 46.2% had other forms of anxieties, and 7.1% exhibited phobic symptoms. Levy and coworkers (1996) found that 40% of patients with MMSE (Folstein et al., 1975) scores between 23 and 26—mild dementia—exhibited depressed symptomatology as elicited by the Alzheimer's Assessment Scale, Non-Cognitive Portion (ADAS-Noncog) (Rosen et al., 1984).

In a sample of 125 patients with AD and MMSE scores above 24 (from the Contact Study) assessed with the Neuropsychiatric Inventory (NPI) (Cummings et al., 1994), depression was found in 44.8% of cases (Table 3–1). The mean scores of affected patients were low (1.5; range of possible scores 0–12), suggesting that while depressive symptoms were common, they were rarely severe. In a sample of normal elderly controls assessed with the NPI (Cummings et al., 1994), the mean score for depression was 0.25, whereas the mean score in the total group of AD patients described above was 1.13. This indicates that depressive symptoms may be present in the normal elderly population, but they occur at substantially lower levels than in mildly impaired AD patients. In the Contact Study, 40% of patients with MMSE scores

Table 3–1. Percentage of Alzheimer's Disease Patients with Mini-Mental State Examination Scores of 25 or Higher, with Symptoms on the Neuropsychiatric Inventory and Mean Score (Range: 0–12) of the Affected Patients ($N = 125$)

Symptom	Percent affected	Mean score of symptomatic patients
Depression	44.8	1.5
Anxiety	40.0	1.7
Irritability	38.4	1.7
Apathy	29.6	2.6
Agitation	28.8	1.4
Aberrant motor behavior	18.4	1.7
Sleep disturbances	16.8	1.1
Appetite changes	15.7	1.3
Disinhibition	11.2	0.5
Delusions	10.4	1.2
Hallucinations	7.2	0.5
Elation	6.4	0.1

Source: Cummings et al. (1994).

of 25 or above exhibited anxiety symptoms, with a mean anxiety subscale score of 1.7 (possible range 0–12).

Thus, reports of anxiety and depression in patients in mild phases of AD suggest that these two symptoms are frequently present even in mildly affected patients. Severe anxiety and depression are not common.

PERSONALITY ALTERATIONS ACCOMPANYING ONSET OF ALZHEIMER'S DISEASE

A variety of types of personality alterations have been described in patients with mild AD. Of these, apathy is the most common. Jost and Grossberg (1996) observed that social withdrawal was the earliest psychiatric symptom exhibited by patients with AD. Among patients with a clinical dementia rating (CDR) (Hughes et al., 1982) of 0.5 (questionable dementia), Rubin and colleagues (1987) found that 6% exhibited diminished emotional responsiveness, 19% had relinquished hobbies, 25% had diminished initiative, and 25% were withdrawn. Of AD patients classified as CDR 1 (mild dementia), 7% had diminished emotional responsiveness, 32% had relinquished hobbies, 39% had diminished initiative, and 23% were withdrawn. These characteristics were elicited using the personality questions of the Blessed Dementia Scale (Blessed et al., 1968).

Siegler and colleagues (1991) used the Neuroticism–Extroversion–Openness to Experience Personality Inventory (NEO) (Costa and McRae, 1985) to assess elderly patients with mild-to-moderate memory impairment, most of whom had AD. The patients were found to have less conscientiousness, lower extroversion, higher neuroticism, and lower openness in their scale profiles. Petry and coworkers (1989), using a personality inventory developed for use in patients with traumatic brain injury (Brooks and McKinlay, 1983), identified a subgroup of patients who exhibited personality alterations early in the course of AD. Nine of the items of the inventory changed in this patient subgroup after disease onset, including being more out of touch, childish, reliant on others, unreasonable, lifeless, cruel, mean, disinterested in company, and quiet.

Self-centeredness is identified as a common personality change in AD patients assessed with the Blessed Dementia scale.

Rubin et al. (1989a,b) found that 5% of normal elderly exhibited this behavior, whereas 34% of patients with questionable dementia and 43% percent of patients with mild dementia were characterized as exhibiting self-centered behavior.

Mega and colleagues (1996) reported personality alterations among patients with mild dementia (MMSE 21–30). They found that 47% were apathetic, 35% were disinhibited, and 35% were irritable. An analysis of patients with AD and MMSE scores of 25 or above (Table 3–1) revealed that 29.6% were apathetic, 11.2% were disinhibited, and 38.4% were irritable. Jost and Grossberg (1996) noted irritability in 50% of patients within 5 months of the diagnosis of AD.

These studies indicate that alterations in personality are common early in the course of AD and are detectable even among patients with very mild alternations in cognition. It is likely that personality alterations are among the earliest changes in behavior to be exhibited by patients with AD.

PSYCHOSIS AS A MANIFESTATION OF EARLY ALZHEIMER'S DISEASE

Delusions or hallucinations can occasionally be the first manifestation of AD. Drevets and Rubin (1989) assessed psychotic symptoms in patients with a CDR scale score of 1 (mild dementia): 30% of the patients had psychotic symptoms; 21% had delusions; 13% had hallucinations; and 12% had misidentification syndromes, including a Capgras-like syndrome (a family member is not who they claim to be), mirror sign (misidentifying one's own reflection in the mirror), and phantom boarder syndrome (unwelcome guests are present in the house). In a study of patients with CDR scores of 0.5 (questionable or very mild dementia), Rubin and coworkers (1993) found that 9% exhibited delusional syndromes, whereas none had misidentification or hallucinations.

Mega and colleagues (1996) reported that 12% of mild AD patients had hallucinations and 12% had delusions. There were no differences in the psychotic symptoms of patients younger than age 64 compared to those at age 65 and above. Among a larger sample ($n = 125$) of AD patients with the MMSE scores of

25 or above studied with the NPI, 10.4% had delusions and 7.2% had hallucinations (Table 3–1). Levy and colleagues (1996) found that 19% of AD patients with MMSE scores between 23 and 26 evidenced psychotic symptoms on the ADAS-Noncog. Jost and Grossberg (1996) observed that 10% of AD patients exhibited delusions within 5 months of the time of diagnosis.

Thus, psychosis, particularly delusional disorders, while less common than mood changes and personality alterations, may occur early in the course of AD, can sometimes be the initial manifestation of the disease, and may occur among patients with mild or very mild dementia syndromes. Few idiopathic psychotic disorders begin late in life, and the occurrence of new-onset psychosis in patients over the age of 60 should arouse consideration of the presence of AD.

AGITATION AS A MANIFESTATION OF EARLY ALZHEIMER'S DISEASE

Agitation is usually considered to be characteristic of the later phases of AD, and it is more prevalent in patients with severe than in those with mild disease (Mega et al., 1996). However, AD patients may have episodes of agitation even when they are only mildly cognitively impaired and in early phases of their illness. Reisberg and colleagues (1989) found that 21.4% of AD patients with a global deterioration scale score of 3 (mild dementia) exhibited purposeless activity such as fidgeting and pacing, 14.3% had verbal outbursts, and 28.6% had nonverbal anger and negativity or other forms of agitation. Levy and colleagues (1996) reported that 38% of AD patients with MMSE scores between 23 and 26 evidenced agitation on the ADAS-Noncog. Mega and co-workers (1996) found that 47% of patients with mild dementia (MMSE scores above 20) had periods of agitation within the 4 weeks preceding interview with the NPI. Among AD patients with MMSE scores of 25 or above assessed with the NPI, 28.8% had periods of agitation within the previous month (Table 3–1).

The few studies that have examined the occurrence of agitation in early AD patients revealed that episodes of agitation are relatively common, occurring in 30% to 40% of patients with mild cognitive impairment.

PATHOPHYSIOLOGY OF NEUROPSYCHIATRIC SYMPTOMS: INSIGHTS FROM NEUROIMAGING

Positron emission tomography (PET) provides insight into the possible pathophysiological basis of early behavioral changes in AD. Minoshima and colleagues (1997) showed reductions in metabolic activity in the posterior cingulate cortex in very early AD. This region has behaviorally relevant reciprocal connections with the prefrontal region, posterior hippocampal areas, and pre-subiculum, as well as receiving afferents from the hippocampus and anterior thalamus and sending efferents to the orbitofrontal area, posterior temporal regions, and dorsal caudate (Mega and Cummings, 1997). There are also reciprocal connections with the frontoparietal region, suggesting that posterior cingulate dysfunction could lead to adverse influences in widespread neocortical and paralimbic regions.

Studying patients with neuropsychiatric symptoms, Sultzer and colleagues (1995) found significant relationships between agitation and reduced metabolism in the frontal and temporal lobes, between psychosis and reduced metabolism in the frontal lobe, and between depression and reduced metabolism in the parietal lobe. Mentis and coworkers (1995) found that AD patients with delusional misidentification syndromes had significantly lower metabolism in orbitofrontal and cingulate areas bilaterally, as well as in the left medial temporal area, compared to AD patients without these symptoms.

Studies using single photon emission computer tomography (SPECT) show reductions in perfusion in the left frontal lobe or left and right temporal lobes (Starkstein et al., 1994; Kotrla et al., 1995) in psychotic compared to nonpsychotic AD patients.

Major depression in AD patients is associated with significantly reduced perfusion in the left superior temporal and parietal regions. Those with major depression also have reduced perfusion of left dorsolateral prefrontal, temporal, and parietal cortices, as well as the right temporal cortex, compared to AD patients with dysthymia (Starkstein et al., 1995).

These metabolic and perfusion studies suggest that patients with neuropsychiatric symptoms represent a neurobiologically distinct subgroup of AD patients with greater involvement of paralimbic and frontal cortex. The early occurrence of these symptoms in patients with minimal cognitive impairment implies that these brain regions are affected earlier and more severely in neuropsychiatrically symptomatic patients.

NEUROBIOLOGY OF NEUROPSYCHIATRIC SYMPTOMS

The neuropathological and neurochemical changes in AD are not global but show regional patterns, and these patterns may relate to the neuropsychiatric symptoms present in patients with mild cognitive impairment. Understandably, studies of the pathology of AD are virtually limited to patients with advanced disease and must be extrapolated with caution to patients in earlier phases of the illness. Zubenko and colleagues (1991) found that psychosis was associated with significantly increased densities of senile plaques and neurofibrillary tangles in the presubiculum and middle frontal cortex, respectively. Psychosis was also associated with the relative preservation of norepinephrine in substantia nigra and a significant reduction of serotonin in the presubiculum.

Victoroff and colleagues (1996) found that AD patients exhibiting physical aggression had greater preservation of pigmented substantia nigra neurons, implying a greater integrity of dopaminergic circuits in aggressive patients.

Palmer and coworkers (1988) found that indoleamines were reduced to 50% to 63% of control values in frontal regions of patients with AD; they speculated that these changes might contribute to the behavioral alterations. This is supported by observations made by Förstl and colleagues (1994), who noted that delusions and hallucinations correlated with lower cell counts in the dorsal raphe nucleus, the origin of serotonergic projections to the cortex.

Perry and colleagues (1990) noted that choline acetyltransferase was significantly more reduced in patients with Lewy body dementia who exhibited hallucinations than in patients who did not have hallucinatory experiences. Lewy body dementia has many of the features of AD. Cummings and Kaufer (1996) hypothesized that the cholinergic disturbance of AD may contribute to many of the behavioral disturbances of AD, including hallucinations, delusions, agitation, apathy, disinhibition, and aberrant motor behavior (pacing, rummaging, etc.).

Lower cell counts in the locus ceruleus of the brain stem have been found in depressed than in nondepressed patients with AD (Zubenko and Moossy, 1988; Zweig et al., 1988; Chan-Palay and Asan, 1989; Förstl et al., 1992). Some investigators also have found reductions in cell counts in the substantia nigra (Zubenko and Moossy, 1988), whereas others have not (Förstl et al., 1992). Zubenko and colleagues (1990) reported marked reductions of norepinephrine in the cortex of depressed patients, compared to nondepressed patients. Serotonin levels were modestly but not significantly lower, and the dopamine levels were higher in the entorhinal cortex of depressed patients with AD. Choline acetyltransferase levels were relatively preserved in subcortical regions of depressed patients.

Using neurofibrillary tangle counts, Braak and Braak (1997) divided AD into transentorhinal stages, limbic stages, and neocortical stages. They observed that in the earliest phases of the illness, tangles appear in the transentorhinal cortex. In the limbic stages of the illness, neurofibrillary tangles are found throughout the paralimbic cortex, including inferior temporal, posterior cingulate, and orbitofrontal regions. In the neocortical stages of the disease, the tangles are found in the paralimbic and heteromodal cortex, with few in the primary sensory and motor regions. Thus, limbic and paralimbic regions are among the earliest brain areas affected in AD, and limbic areas are known to mediate important aspects of emotional activity.

These studies indicate that there are regional differences in the severity of neuropathological and neurochemical changes in patients with neuropsychiatric symptoms compared to those without. Assuming that these changes can be extrapolated back to the initial phases of the illness, it is likely that there are regional differences in the neuropathologic burden and neurochemical alterations in neuropsychiatrically symptomatic patients with minimal cognitive impairment. These changes might reflect differences in the distribution of the pathology in specific subtypes of AD or individual differences in the susceptibility of neurons in various brain regions.

ASSESSMENT OF NEUROPSYCHIATRIC SYMPTOMS IN ALZHEIMER'S DISEASE

Neuropsychiatric symptoms are a common feature of AD (Reisberg et al., 1987; Mega et al., 1996) and, as shown in this survey of the literature, behavioral symptoms may be present early in the disease. Neuropsychiatric symptoms are an important cause of caregiver distress (Kaufer et al., 1998) and are amenable to treatment with cholinergic agents or conventional psychotropic drugs (Cummings, 2002). Early detection of AD based on these symptoms would allow early treatment with agents that slow progression of the disease—agents such as vitamin E and selegiline. The observation that the neuropsychiatric symptoms sometimes precede the onset of cognitive impairment implies that detection of these symptoms would identify patients at high risk for developing AD and might be a means of recognizing one subgroup of AD patients at an earlier time than cognitive assessments currently allow.

There is an urgent need to identify patients with AD in minimally symptomatic stages of the illness, and an awareness of the neuropsychiatric presentations of AD and recognition of the importance of screening for these disturbances may have important public health consequences. Physicians and family members who might ascribe behavioral changes to normal aging must be made cognizant of the potential importance of these symptoms as markers of early AD.

Effective screening methodologies for the detection and characterization of neuropsychiatric symptoms in early AD must also be developed and distributed. Complex, time-consuming rating scales and inventories are not likely to gain widespread application. Simple symptom checklists are preferable if they can be made sufficiently sensitive to detect the major early neuropsychiatric symptoms. Use of multidimensional rating scales is of obvious importance, given the wide range of neuropsychiatric symptoms that may occur in early AD. Instruments such as the NPI (Cummings et al., 1994), Behave AD (Reisberg et al., 1987), and the Behavior Rating Scale for Dementia (Tariot et al., 1995) are examples of multidimensional rating scales that assay a broad range of neuropsychiatric symptoms. They do not address concomitant cognitive alterations or changes in functional abilities.

Combining a behavioral assessment with biological markers may increase the positive predictive value of behavioral changes in late life for the development of AD. For example, the combination of apathy or irritability with an *APOE-4* genotype may have substantially greater predictive value than the occurrence of apathy or irritability alone. Similarly, medial temporal lobe atrophy revealed by magnetic resonance imaging or computerized tomography in a patient who also exhibits neuropsychiatric symptoms (depression, irritability, apathy, anxiety) may predict the occurrence of AD with much greater accuracy than either finding alone. Since the neuropsychiatric changes likely reflect the presence of the AD process—although not yet sufficiently intense or distributed to produce major cognitive impairment—the neurobiological correlates of AD-type pathology, such as reduced β-amyloid or increased tau protein in the cerebrospinal fluid, might also be present in neuropsychiatrically symptomatic patients and predictive of ensuing cognition impairment.

The occurrence of neuropsychiatric symptoms as common features of early AD suggests that they can be followed in the course of clinical trials. Disturbances such as apathy that correlate highly with cognitive impairment and increase regularly across the course of the disease with relatively little fluctuation readily lend themselves to inclusion in clinical trials as measures of disease severity. Others, such as depression, psychosis, and agitation, are more episodic, although they generally increase in the course of the disease. These fluctuating symptoms require different analytic strategies to detect the effect of disease interventions. The consistent emergence of new psychiatric symptoms during the course of the illness suggests that the delay of emergence of new symptoms may be an effective analytical approach sensitive to disease interventions that affect the progression of AD.

SUMMARY

In summary, neuropsychiatric symptoms are part of the clinical syndrome of AD in many patients with minimal cognitive impairment. Assessment of these symptoms may increase sensitivity for the early detection of AD and may provide novel measures to detect the impact of interventions that slow disease progression.

Acknowledgments

This work was supported by a National Institute on Aging Alzheimer's Disease Center grant (AG 10123) and the Sidell-Kagan Foundation.

References

Agbayewa, M.O. (1986). Earlier psychiatric morbidity in patients with Alzheimer's disease. *J Am Geriatr Soc* 34:561–564.

Agency for Health Care Policy and Research. (1996). Early Alzheimer's Disease: Recognition and Assessment. Washington, DC: U.S. Department of Health and Human Services.

Alexopoulos, G.S., B.S. Meyers, R.C. Young, S. Mattis, and T. Kakuma. (1993). The course of Geriatric Depression with "reversible dementia": a controlled study. *Am J Psychiatry* 150:1693–1699.

Baker, F.M., E. Kokmen, V. Chandra, and B.S. Schoenberg. (1991). Psychiatric symptoms in cases of clinically diagnosed Alzheimer's disease. *J Geriatr Psychiatry Neurol* 4:71–78.

Blessed, G., B.E. Tomlinson, and M. Roth. (1968). The association between quantitative measures of dementia and of senile changes in the cerebral grey matter of elderly subjects. *Br J Psychol* 225:797–811.

Braak, H., and E. Braak. (1997). Aspects of cortical destruction in Alzheimer's disease. In Connections, Cognition, and Alzheimer's Disease, edited by B.T. Hyman, C. Duyckaerts, and Y. Christen. Frankfurt, Germany: Springer-Verlag.

Broe, G.A., A.S. Henderson, H. Creasey, E. McCusker, A.E. Korten, A.F. Jorm, W. Longley, and J.C. Anthony. (1990). A case-control study of Alzheimer's disease in Australia. *Neurology* 40:1698–1707.

Brooks, D.N., and W. McKinlay. (1983). Personality and behavior changes after severe blunt head injury: a relative's view. *J Neurol Neurosurgery Psychiatry* 46:336–344.

Caine, E.D. (1981). Pseudodementia: current concepts and future directions. *Arch General Psychiatry* 38:1359–1364.

Chan-Palay, V., and E. Asan. (1989). Alterations in catecholamine neurons of the locus coeruleus in senile dementia of the Alzheimer type and in Parkinson's disease with and without dementia and depression. *J Comparative Neurol* 287:373–392.

Corder, E.H., A.M. Saunders, W.J. Strittmatter, D.E. Schmechel, P.C. Gaskell, G.W. Small, A.D. Roses, J.L. Haines, and M.A. Pericak-Vance. (1993). Gene dose of apoliproprotein E type 4 allele and the risk of Alzheimer's disease in late onset families. *Science* 261:921–923.

Costa, P.T., and R.R. McCrae. (1985). The NEO Personality Inventory. Los Angeles: Western Psychological Services.

Crystal, H.A., L.I. Wolfson, and S. Ewing. (1988). Visual hallucinations as the first symptom of Alzheimer's disease. *Am J Psychiatry* 145:10.

Cummings, J.L. (2002). Neuropsychiatry of Alzheimer's disease and related disorders. London: Martin Dunitz.

Cummings, J.L. (1989). Dementia and depression: an evolving enigma. *J Neuropsychiatry Clin Neurosci* 1:236–242.

Cummings, J.L., and D. Kaufer. (1996). Neuropsychiatric aspects of Alzheimer's disease: the cholinergic hypothesis revisited. *Neurology* 47:876–883.

Cummings, J.L., M. Mega, K. Gray, S. Rosenberg-Thompson, D.A. Carusi, and J. Gornbein. (1994). The Neuropsychiatric Inventory: comprehensive assessment of psychopathology in dementia. *Neurology* 44:2308–2314.

Cummings, J.L., H.V. Vinters, G.M. Cole, and Z.S. Khachaturian. (1998). Alzheimer's disease: etiologies, pathophysiology, cognitive reserve, and treatment opportunities. *Neurology* 51(suppl.):S2–S17.

Devanand, D.P., M. Sano, T. Ming-Xin, S. Taylor, B.J. Gurland, D. Wilder, Y. Stern, and R. Mayeux. (1996). Depressed mood and the incidence of Alzheimer's disease in the elderly living in the community. *Arch General Psychiatry* 53:175–182.

Drevets, W.C., and E.H. Rubin. (1989). Psychotic symptoms and the longitudinal course of senile dementia of the Alzheimer type. *Biological Psychiatry* 25:39–48.

Folstein, M.F., S.E. Folstein, and P.R. McHugh. (1975). The "mini-mental state": a practical method for grading the cognitive state of patients for the clinician. *J Psychiatric Res* 12:189–198.

Förstl, H., A. Burns, P. Luthert, N. Cairns, P. Lantos, and R. Levy. (1992). Clinical and neuropathological correlates of depression in Alzheimer's disease. *Psychol Med* 22:877–884.

Förstl, H., A. Burns, R. Levy, and N. Cairns. (1994). Neuropathological correlates of psychotic phenomena in confirmed Alzheimer's disease. *Br J Psychiatry* 165:53–59.

Förstl, H., R. Zerfaß, C. Geiger-Kabisch, H. Sattel, C. Besthorn, and F. Hentschel. (1995). Brain atrophy in normal aging and Alzheimer's disease volumetric discrimination and clinical correlations. *Br J Psychiatry* 167:739–746.

French, L.R., L.M. Schuman, J.A. Mortimer, J.T. Hutton, R.A. Boatman, and B. Christians. (1985). A case-control study of dementia of the Alzheimer type. *Am J Epidemiol* 121:414–421.

Haxby, J.V., C.L. Grady, R. Durara, N. Schlageter, G. Berg, and S.I. Rapoport. (1986). Neocortical metabolic abnormalities precede non-memory cognitive defects in early Alzheimer's-type dementia. *Arch Neurol* 43:882–885.

Heidrich A., J. Thome, and M. Rosler. (1997). Apolipoprotein E-e4 frequency in late-onset depression. *Biol Psychiatry* 41:912–914.

Hughes, C.P., L. Berg, W.L. Danziger, L.A. Coben, and R.L. Martin. (1982). A new clinical scale for the staging of dementia. *Br J Psychiatry* 140:566–572.

Jobst, K.A., A.D. Smith, M. Szatmari, A. Molyneux, M.M. Esiri, E. King, A. Smith, A. Jaskowski, B. McDonald, and N. Wald. (1992a). Detection in life of confirmed Alzheimer's disease using a simple measurement of medical temporal lobe atrophy computed by tomography. *Lancet* 340:1179–1183.

Jobst, K.A., A.D. Smith, C.S. Barker, A. Wear, E.M. King, A. Smith, P.A. Anslow, A.J. Molyneux, B.J. Shepstone, N. Soper, K.A. Holmes, J.R. Robinson, R.A. Hope, C. Oppenheimer, K. Brockbank, and B. McDonald. (1992b). Association of atrophy of the medial temporal lobe with reduced blood flow in the posterior parietotemporal cortex in patients with a clinical and pathological diagnosis of Alzheimer's disease. *J Neurol Neurosurgery Psychiatry* 55:190-194.

Jost, B.C., and G.T. Grossberg. (1996). The evolution of psychiatric symptoms in Alzheimer's disease: a natural history study. *J Am Geriatr Soc* 44: 1078–1081.

Kaufer, D.I., J.L. Cummings, D. Christine, T. Bray, S. Castellon, A. Macmillan, P. Ketchel, and D. Masterman. (1998). The impact of neuropsychiatric symptoms in Alzheimer's disease: the neuropsychiatric inventory caregiver distress scale. *J Am Geriatr Soc* 46:210–215.

Kokmen, E., C.M. Beard, V. Chandra, K.P. Offord, B.S. Schoenberg, and D.J. Ballard (1991). Clinical risk factors for Alzheimer's disease: a population-based case-control study. *Neurology* 41:1393–1397.

Kotrla, K.J., C.C. Ranjit, R.G. Harper, S. Jhingran, and R. Doody. (1995). SPECT findings on psychosis in Alzheimer's disease. *Am J Psychiatry* 152. 1470–1475.

Kral, V.A., and O.B. Emery. (1989). Long-term follow-up of depressive pseudodementia of the aged. *Can J Psychiatry* 34:445–446.

Krishnan, K.R.R., L.A. Tupler, J.C. Ritchie, W.M. McDonald, D.L. Knight, C.B. Nemeroff, and B.J. Carroll. (1996). Apolipoprotein E-e4 frequency in geriatric depression. *Biological Psychiatry* 40:69–71.

La Rue, A., J. Spar, and C. Dessonville-Hill. (1986). Cognitive impairment in late-life depression: clinical correlates and treatment implications. *J Affect Disorders* 11:179–184.

Lesser, I.M., B.L. Miller, K.B. Boone, E. Hill-Gutierrez, and I. Mena. (1989). Psychosis as the first manifestation of degenerative dementia. Bull Clin Neurosci 54:59–63.

Levy, M.I., J.L. Cummings, L.A. Fairbanks, D. Bravi, M. Calvani, and A. Carta. (1996). Longitudinal assessment of symptoms of depression, agitation, and psychosis in 181 patients with Alzheimer's disease. *Am J Psychiatry* 153:1438–1443.

Liston, E.H. Jr. (1977). Occult presenile dementia. *J Nervous Mental Dis* 164: 263–267.

McHugh, P.R., and M.F. Folstein. (1979). Psychopathology of dementia: implications for neuropathology. In Congenital and Acquired Cognitive Disorders, edited by R. Katzman (pp. 17–30). New York: Raven Press.

Mega, M.S., and J.L. Cummings. (1997). The cingulate and cingulate syndromes. In Contemporary Behavioral Neurology, edited by M.R. Trimble and J.L. Cummings (pp. 189–214). Boston: Butterworth-Heinemann.

Mega, M.S., J.L. Cummings, T. Fiorello, and J. Gornbein. (1996). The spectrum of behavioral changes in Alzheimer's disease. *Neurology* 46:130–135.

Mentis, M.J., E.A. Weinstein, B. Horwitz, A.R. McIntosh, P. Pietrini, G.E. Alexander, M. Furey, and D.G.M. Murphy. (1995). Abnormal brain glucose metabolism in the delusional misidentification syndromes: a positron emission tomography study in Alzheimer disease. *Biol Psychiatry* 38:438–449.

Minoshima, S., B. Giordani, S. Berent, K.A. Frey, N.L. Foster, and D.E. Kuhl. (1997). Metabolic reduction in the posterior cingulate cortex in very early Alzheimer's disease. *Ann Neurol* 42:85–94.

Palmer, A.M., G.C. Stratmann, A.W. Procter, and D.M. Bowen. (1988). Possible neurotransmitter basis of behavioral changes in Alzheimer's disease. *Ann Neurol* 23:616–620.

Parks, R.W., and R.F. Zec. (1993). Neuropsychological functioning in Alzheimer's disease. In *Neuropsychology of Alzheimer's Disease and Other Dementias*, edited by R.S. Wilson (pp. 3–80). New York: Oxford University Press.

Pearlson, G.D., P.V. Rabins, W.S. Kim, L.J. Speedie, P.J. Moberg, A. Burns, and M.J. Bascom. (1989). Structural brain CT changes and cognitive deficits in elderly depressives with and without reversible dementia ("pseudodementia"). *Psychol Med* 19:573–584.

Perry, E.K., J. Kerwin, R.H. Perry, D. Irving, G. Blessed, and A. Fairbairn. (1990). Cerebral cholinergic activity is related to the incidence of visual hallucinations in senile dementia of Lewy body type. *Dementia* 1:2–4.

Petry, S., J.L. Cummings, M. Hill, and J. Shapira. (1989). Personality alterations in dementia of the Alzheimer type: a three-year follow-up study. *J Geriatr Psychiatry Neurol* 4:203–207.

Rabins, P.V., A. Merchant, and G. Nestadt. (1984). Criteria for diagnosing reversible dementia caused by depression: validation by 2-year follow-up. *Br J Psychiatry* 144:488–492.

Reisberg, B., J. Borenstein, S.P. Salob, S.H. Ferris, E. Franssen, and A. Georotas. (1987). Behavioral symptoms in Alzheimer's disease: phenomenology and treatment. *J Clin Psychiatry* 48(5, Suppl.):9–15.

Reisberg, B., E. Franssen, S.G. Sclan, A. Kluger, and S. Ferris. (1989). Stage specific incidence of potentially remediable behavioral symptoms in aging and Alzheimer disease: a study of 120 patients using the BEHAVE-AD. *Bull Clin Neurosci* 54:95–112.

Rosen, W.G., R.C. Mohs, and K.L. Davis. (1984). A new rating rule for Alzheimer's disease. *Am J Psychiatry* 141:1356–1364.

Rubin, E.H., J.C. Morris, M. Storandt, and L. Berg. (1987). Behavioral changes in patients with mild senile dementia of the Alzheimer's type. *Psychiatry Res* 21:55–62.

Rubin, E.H., D.A. Kinscherf, and J.C. Morris. (1989a). Personality and dementia. *Bull Clin Neurosci* 54:88–94.

Rubin, E.H., D.A. Kinscherf, and J.C. Morris. (1989b). Psychopathology of very mild dementia of the Alzheimer type. *Am J Psychiatry* 146:1017–1021.

Rubin, E.H, D.A. Kinscherf, and J.C. Morris. (1993). Psychopathology in younger versus older persons with very mild and mild dementia of the Alzheimer type. *Am J Psychiatry* 150:639–642.

Sachdev, P.S., J.S. Smith, H. Angus-Lepan, and P. Rodriguez. (1990). Pseudodementia twelve years on. *J Neurol Neurosurgery Psychiatry* 53:254–259.

Shalat, S.L., B. Seltzer, C. Pidcock, and E.L. Baker Jr. (1987). Risk factors for Alzheimer's disease: a case-control study. *Neurology* 37:1630-1633.

Siegler, I.C., K.A. Welsh, D.V. Dawson, G.G. Fillenbaum, N.L. Earl, E.B. Kaplan, and C.M. Clark. (1991). Ratings of personality change in patients being evaluated for memory disorders. *Alzheimer Dis Assoc Disorders* 5:240–250.

Starkstein, S.E., S. Vásquez, G. Petracca, L. Sabe, R. Migliorelli, A. Tesón, and R. Leiguarda. (1994). A SPECT study of delusions in Alzheimer's disease. *Neurology* 44:2055–2059.

Starkstein, S.E., S. Vásquez, R. Migliorelli, A. Tesón, G. Petracca, and R. Leiguarda. (1995). A SPECT study of depression in Alzheimer's disease. *Neuropsychiatry, Neuropsychol Behav Neurol* 8:38–43.

Steffens, D.C., B.L. Plassman, M.J. Helms, K.A. Welsh-Bohmer, A.M. Saunders, and C.S. Breitner. (1997). A twin study of late-onset depression and apolipoprotein E-e4 as risk factors for Alzheimer's disease. *Biol Psychiatry* 41:851–856.

Sultzer, D.L., M.E. Mahler, M.A. Mandelkern, J.L. Cummings, W.G. Van Gorp, C.H. Hinkin, and M.A. Berisford. (1995). The relationship between psychiatric symptoms and regional cortical metabolism in Alzheimer's disease. *J Neuropsychiatry Clin Neurosci* 7:476–484.

Tariot, P.N., J.L. Jack, M.B. Patterson, S.D. Edland, M.F. Weiner, G. Fillenbaum, L. Blazina, L. Teri, E. Rubin, J.A. Mortimer, Y. Stern, and the Behavioral Pathology Committee of the Consortium to Establish a Registry for Alzheimer's Disease. (1995). The behavior rating scale for dementia of the Consortium to Establish a Registry for Alzheimer's Disease. *Am J Psychiatry* 152:1349–1357.

Victoroff, J., C. Zarow, W.J. Mack, E. Hsu, and H.C. Chui. (1996). Physical aggression is associated with preservation of substantia nigra pars compacta in Alzheimer disease. *Arch Neurol* 53:428–434.

Wands, K., D.M. Merskey, V.V. Hachinski, M. Fishman, H. Fox, and M. Boniferro. (1990). A questionnaire investigation of anxiety and depression in early dementia. *J Am Geriatr Soc* 38:535–538.

Wells, C.E. (1979). Pseudodementia. *Am J Psychiatry* 136:895–900.

Zubenko, G.S., and J. Moossy. (1988). Major depression in primary dementia: Clinical and neuropathologic correlates. *Arch Neurol* 45:1182–1186.

Zubenko, G.S., J. Moossy, and U. Kopp. (1990). Neurochemical correlates of major depression in primary dementia. *Arch Neurol* 47:209–214.

Zubenko, G.S., J. Moossy, A.J. Martinez, G. Rao, D. Claassen, J. Rosen, and U. Kopp. (1991). Neuropathologic and neurochemical correlates of psychosis in primary dementia. *Arch Neurol* 48:619–624.

Zubenko, G.S., R. Henderson, J.S. Stiffler, S. Stabler, J. Rosen, and B. Kaplan. (1996). Association of the apo E4 allele with clinical subtypes of late life depression. *Biol Psychiatry* 40:1008–1016.

Zweig, R.M., C.A. Ross, J.C. Hedreen, C. Steele, J.E. Cardillo, P.J. Whitehouse, M.F. Folstein, and D.L. Price. (1988). The neuropathology of aminergic nuclei in Alzheimer's disease. *Ann Neurol* 24:233–242.

CHAPTER 4

Normative Neuropsychology

GLENN E. SMITH
ROBERT J. IVNIK

The ability to distinguish categories along the continuum from normal aging to disease is enhanced by neuropsychological assessment. In turn, the usefulness of neuropsychological assessment is enhanced by normative neuropsychological research to establish the psychometric properties of neuropsychological instruments. The Mayo Older Americans Normative Studies (MOANS) were undertaken to provide age-appropriate norms up to life's oldest ages. In the conduct of these studies several guiding principals have been employed. A model of typical aging was used to define "normal." Co-norming and longitudinal methods were used to enhance the ability to compare cognitive performances at a single point in time and across time. Statistical analyses emphasized the provision of clinically useful, "individual" statistics to supplement group analyses. An attempt has been made to employ sound epidemiological principles. We hope that these efforts contribute to the ability to identify mild cognitive impairment (MCI) as a condition with high risk for subsequent development of dementia.

NEED FOR NEUROPSYCHOLOGICAL NORMS

In 1984 and 1986, two documents were published which were of great relevance to the spectrum from normal functioning to disease. First, NINCDS-ADRDA (McKhann et al., 1984) criteria were published for the diagnosis of Alzheimer's disease (AD). The document providing these diagnostic criteria for AD noted that neuropsychological test data were of value in confirming the requisite presence of dementia for the purposes of diagnosing AD. However, the document also noted that "there are no normative population standards for many of these tests" (McKhann et al., 1984, p. 941). Implicit in this commentary was the notion that cognitive changes of dementia are distinct from normal cognitive aging and more needed to be known about normal older persons' performance on neuropsychological measures for psychometric measures to help distinguish these differences.

Then an NIMH work group published provisional criteria for the diagnosis of age-associated memory impairment (AAMI) (Crook et al., 1986). These criteria were intended to establish a diagnostic entity that could be applied in persons whose complaints involved normal age-related changes in cognitive function. These criteria are listed in Table 4–1. Key provisions of these criteria were *(1)* the presence of a subjective memory complaint and *(2)* statistical deviation in memory performance of older adults relative to norms for persons aged 20 to 35. Smith et al. (1991) provided one critique of these diagnostic criteria. They noted that the criteria were underspecified with respect to memory performance. They demonstrated that rates of AAMI in a large sample of normals could vary from 11% to 98%, depending on the use of one versus multiple memory tests and the sensitivity of those memory tests to age-related changes in cognitive function (Smith et al., 1991).

A second area of criticism (Smith et al., 1991; Caine, 1993) related to the wisdom of having a diagnosis for a normal aging process. Different perspectives on whether or not to diagnose age-related changes may relate to underlying conceptual models about aging.

MODELS OF AGING

Biological models of development often distinguish two phases of life: growth and aging. These models are based primarily on the observation that for most organisms there is a period of physical growth and differentiation leading to maturity, then a period

Table 4–1. Proposed Criteria for the Diagnosis of Age-Associated Memory Impairment, National Institute of Mental Health Work Group

Inclusion Criteria

Adults at least 50 years of age

Complaints of memory loss reflected in everyday problems; onset of memory loss described as gradual, no sudden worsening

Memory test performance that is at least 1 SD below the mean established for young adults on a standardized and adequately normed test of secondary (recent) memory; examples of tests and cutoffs provided by the National Institute of Mental Health work group:

- Benton Visual Retention Test (Form A)—6 or fewer correct
- Wechsler Memory Scale, Logical Memory subtest—6 or fewer correct
- Wechsler Memory Scale, Associate Learning subtest—13 or fewer correct

Evidence of adequate intellectual function reflected in a standard score of at least 9 on the Wechsler Adult Intelligence Scale

Absence of dementia reflected in a score of 24 or higher on the Mini-Mental State Exam

Exclusion Criteria

Evidence of delirium, confusion, or other disturbances of consciousness

Presence of any neurological disorder determined by history, clinical neurological examination, or neuroradiographic examination that could produce cognitive deterioration

History of infective or inflammatory brain disease

Evidence of significant cerebral vascular pathology as determined by a Hachinski ischemia score of 4 or more

History of repeated minor head injury or single head injury with greater than 1 hr loss of consciousness

Current psychiatric diagnosis of depression, mania, or major psychiatric diagnosis

Current diagnosis or history of alcohol or drug dependence

Evidence of depression as determined by a Hamilton Rating Scale for Depression score of 13 or more

Any medical disorder determined by history, clinical examination, and laboratory tests that could produce cognitive deterioration

Psychotropic drug use during the month before psychometric testing

Source: From T. Crook, R.T. Bartus, S.H. Ferris, P. Whitehouse, G.D. Cohen, and S. Gershon (1986). Age associated memory impairment: proposed diagnostic criteria and measures of clinical change—report of a National Institute of Mental Health Work Group, *Developmental Neuropsychology* 2:270–271. Copyright 1986 by Lawrence Erlbaum. Adapted by permission.

of senescing (Schroots and Birren, 1996). "Senescing" refers to a loss of functional capacity and adaptability. The AAMI diagnostic criteria seem to arise from a biological model of aging. This is especially evident in the requirement that older adults' memory performances be compared to 20- to 34-year-old norms. Cross-sectional data on memory performance suggest this is the age of optimal or "mature" memory function (Albert, 1988). As diseases also produce loss of functional capacity and adaptability, aging and disease are often viewed in parallel in biological aging.

A contrasting view is the life-span development perspective (Baltes and Reese, 1984) which has arisen in part from the psychology of aging field. Within this perspective, "the changes (growth, development, aging) shown by people from the time of their conception, throughout their lives, and until the time of their death are usefully conceptualized as development" (Baltes and Reese, 1984, p. 493). Within this model, "maturation" continues after physical growth, continuing even until the time of death. Throughout maturation, psychological processes change. The life-span development perspective recognizes changing functional status as a characteristic of the individual throughout life and avoids terms that suggest abnormality for these processes.

These contrasting views of aging may lead to different conclusions about intervening with age-related changes, although such conclusions are not mandated by the different models. A biological aging or senescence model may lead to the conclusion that age-related changes, like disease symptoms, need to be diagnosed so treatment can be prescribed. The condition of presbycusis provides a good example of this model. Accurate identification of common, age-related changes in hearing can lead to provision of hearing aids, which maintain functional independence. A life-span perspective is less likely to view age-related cognitive changes as a "condition" and more as a "stage of life." The response to this stage may be to change our expectations for the person, rather than change the person. Retirement provides a good example of a life-span development "intervention." Retirement is typically seen as a developmental phase rather than as "work impairment."

Whether researchers and clinicians embrace a senescence or life-span development model of aging will importantly influence their approach to the spectrum from normal aging to disease. Advocates of one or another model of aging will embrace different definitions of normal aging, which will influence their approaches to normative neuropsychology. It should be recognized that choices about models of aging and definitions of normal aging are not typically determined on an empiric basis. Rather, these choices reflect philosophical decisions that must be made by researchers and clinicians.

DEFINITIONS OF NORMAL AGING

Models of aging influence definitions of normal aging. Experimental neuropsychologists and cognitive-aging researchers endeavor to study the affects of aging alone on cognitive function. The definition of aging as the passage of time alone, exclusive of age-related diseases, has been associated with the term "successful aging" (Rowe and Kahn, 1987). Within this paradigm, older persons with common medical illnesses that have the slightest potential to affect cognition (e.g., diabetes or chronic obstructive pulmonary disease) are excluded from study. Similarly, patients taking medications that might influence cognition (e.g., beta blockers) are also excluded from study. This enables cognitive-aging theorists to isolate the effect of the passage of time alone on the organism's cognition. Cohorts of persons studied in these paradigms are often described as "super normals" because their performances tend to cluster at the upper end of the distribution of cognitive functioning. Studies of successful aging provide a picture of the effect of uncomplicated yet uncommon forms of aging on cognitive function.

An alternate approach in cognitive-aging studies is to study typical aging. Within this definition of normal aging, persons with common medical conditions, using common medications, and the like, are not excluded from study. This definition accepts common age-associated diseases as physiologically typical of the aging process—that is, part of development. Studies of typical aging often provide a different and perhaps less optimistic picture of normal cognitive aging than do studies of optimal aging (LaRue, 1992; Powell, 1994).

However, studies of typical aging are of special value to clinicians who practice in settings where they must distinguish neuropathology-related cognitive impairment (e.g., dementias and deliriums) from other age-related processes. For these clinicians, the representativeness of the cognitive aging cohort under study compared to the typical clinical patient is of great importance. So, typical aging is perhaps the definition of normal aging most embraced in normative studies of aging. Admittedly, normative studies of aging have a different focus than do cognitive-aging studies. Whereas the latter seek to define what is possible or common in aging, the goal of the normative studies of aging is "the development of psychometric normative data that are maximally useful in identifying abnormal cognitive function in the elderly" (Malec et al., 1993, p. 81).

COGNITIVE AGING AND NORMATIVE NEUROPSYCHOLOGY

A review of the extensive research and theorizing on cognitive aging, as well as the controversies over the fundamental processes in cognitive aging, are well beyond the scope of this chapter and the scope of normative neuropsychology. These controversies have been discussed elsewhere (e.g., LaRue, 1992). Suffice it to say, there is some consensus that typical cognitive aging appears to involve a loss in efficiency in the acquisition of new information (LaRue, 1992; Petersen et al., 1992). In addition, typical cognitive aging, and perhaps optimal cognitive aging, also involve loss of processing speed, cognitive flexibility, and working memory efficiency (LaRue, 1992). The normative neuropsychology framework focused on typical aging has contributed to the identification of cognitive domains that are relatively spared, even in typical aging, but may be associated with neurological disease states. Among these are access to remotely learned information, including the integrity of the semantic network (Monsch et al., 1994) and the retention of well-encoded new information (Petersen et al., 1992). The latter two of these cognitive processes (delayed recall or retention and use of semantic networks) may be especially sensitive indicators of an early disease process (Masur et al., 1994; Monsch et al., 1994; Petersen et al., 1994; Welsh et al., 1991). This is an example of the utility of normative neuropsychology. By focusing on what is uncommon versus common in typical aging, normative neuropsychology has provided performance referents that highlight neurological disease "signals" while dampening the "noise" of age-related variance in cognitive function.

SUBJECTIVE MEMORY COMPLAINT OR OBJECTIVE MEMORY FUNCTION

If patient complaint were a reliable predictor of memory impairment, the need for standardized memory assessment and appropriate norms would be minimized. In fact, by including the presence of subjective memory complaint in the criteria for AAMI (Crook et al., 1986) (see Table 4–1), authors of those criteria seemed to suggest that such complaints might be a good indictor of functionally significant cognitive compromise. However, several studies have suggested otherwise (Kahn et al., 1975; Plotkin et al., 1985; Larrabee and Levin, 1986; O'Connor et al., 1989; McGlone et al., 1990; Bolla et al., 1991; Taylor et al., 1992; Hanninen et al., 1994). In one study, memory complaint, mood, and longitudinal memory scores were obtained for 294 participants, aged 55 to 97 years. In multiple-regression modeling, mood and current memory scores contributed 20% and 3%, respectively, to subjective memory complaint variance. Longitudinal memory change scores were not associated with the subjective memory scores. This suggested that emotional status or sense of self-efficacy was a better predictor of subjective memory ratings than was either absolute objective memory performance or objective longitudinal memory change (Smith et al., 1996). Persons who developed cognitive impairment over the longitudinal interval in this study did report greater memory problems, but memory complaints had little positive predictive value in identifying these persons. This study was consistent with other reports (Kahn et al., 1975; Plotkin et al., 1985; Larrabee and Levin, 1986; O'Connor et al., 1989; McGlone et al., 1990; Bolla et al., 1991; Taylor et al., 1992; Hanninen et al., 1994) in demonstrating that subjective memory complaint is poorly related to the presence of poor memory performance in cohorts of typical older adults. Since self-reported memory complaint appears more related to affective status or general self-efficacy assessments, they cannot serve as an adequate surrogate for objective memory assessment.

Informant-based reports of memory decline do appear to have an association with objectively measured memory impairments (McGlone et al., 1990). However, one-third to one-half of dementia patients may be residing alone at onset or diagnosis of cognitive impairment (Smith et al., 2000). As such, a reliable informant may routinely be unavailable to report memory decline. The need for objective memory assessment to detect memory impairment may be unavoidable. Since objective assessment seems necessary to reliably establish the presence of memory problems, the problem of adequate norms for such assessments persists, as identified by the NINCDS-ADRDA diagnosis group (McKhann et al., 1984).

MOANS METHODS

The Mayo Older American Normative Studies (MOANS) were initiated in the late 1980s (Ivnik et al., 1992b) to address, in part, the absence of appropriate neuropsychological norms for assessment of older adults. These projects were initiated by clinicians who felt typical aging models are most useful for routine clinical practice. The definition of "normal" selected for these studies was intended to produce a sample of typical older adults. The criteria for normal in the MOANS studies are listed in Table 4–2. Normative data for persons age 75 and younger were generally present on tests targeted in the MOANS studies. Persons aged 55 to 74 were nevertheless intentionally included in the MOANS cohort. This enabled assessment of differences be-

Table 4–2. Mayo Older Americans Normative Studies (MOANS): Criteria for Normal for Persons Aged 55 and Over

No active psychiatric or neurological disease

No complaint of cognitive difficulty during history taking and systems review, and no finding on physical examination suggesting disorders with potential to affect cognition

No psychotropic medication use in amounts that would compromise cognition or suggest neuropsychiatric disorder

Independent community dwelling status

Prior history of disorders (e.g., alcohol abuse) with potential to affect cognition were not automatically excluded as long as the disorder was not active and there was recovery without apparent cognitive residual

Chronic medical illness not exclusionary as long as condition was not reported by physician to compromise cognition

Source: Ivnik et al. (1992a).

tween the MOANS subjects selection process and national normative samples on tests such as the Wechsler Adult Intelligence
Scale–Revised (Wechsler, 1981).

Data collected on the original MOANS sample of 397 patients (Ivnik et al., 1992b) were used to establish norms on the
WAIS-R, the Wechsler Memory Scale–Revised (WMS-R) (Wechsler, 1987), and the Auditory Verbal Learning Test (AVLT) (Rey,
1964). As noted, for the cohort of patients aged 55 to 74, valid
WAIS-R indices could be established. In the MOANS cohort a
mean IQ score of roughly 106 and a standard deviation (SD) of
approximately 11 were observed for this age group. Thus, it was
felt that sample selection in these studies produced a sample of
patients with IQ scores roughly 6 points higher than the national
average of 100, and with less variance than the expected 15-point
SD. It was assumed that similar selection and demographic factors would be operating in the 75 to 97 age range. This is the
age group from whom prior norms did not exist. When norms
were developed for this group, the mean was set at 106, and the
SD at 11 points. To ensure a normal distribution, the frequency
distribution of the raw scores was converted to standard scores
by assigning raw scores at a given percentile to the appropriate
scaled score at the same percentile in the normal curve. The
MOANS procedure also adopted use of overlapping interval
strategies (Pauker, 1988) to maximize the number of subjects
contributing to the normative distribution at each mid-point age
interval. Each successive 3-year age point was used as a mid-point
age interval; and, all subjects, plus or minus 5 years of that age,
were used to establish the distribution for that age group. The
method of overlapping intervals is illustrated in Figure 4–1.

Co-Norming

The MOANS studies were undertaken to co-norm commonly
used neuropsychological tests for persons up to 97 years of age.
Co-norming is the process of simultaneously obtaining data on
multiple tests for the same normative cohort. Co-norming has
multiple advantages. One advantage is affording the opportunity
to establish norms for comparisons among different test scores.
Another advantage is permitting determination of the underlying factor structure of the collection of tests administered together as a battery. After WAIS-R, WMS-R, and AVLT norms for

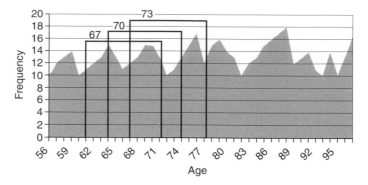

Figure 4–1. Overlapping intervals for normative data: each successive 3-year age point is used as a midpoint age interval, and all subjects, plus or minus 5 years of that age, are used to establish the distribution for that age group. Thus a person who is 70 would contribute to the norms for 67, 70, and 73 midpoint age groups.

persons 55 to 97 (Ivnik et al., 1992a) were developed, co-norming with a variety of other neuropsychological tests was undertaken (Ivnik et al., 1996; Lucas et al., 1998a, 1998b). In addition, the factor structure of the WAIS-R, WMS-R, and AVLT, administered as a battery, was established. Smith and colleagues showed that five cognitive constructs best described the factor structure of the AVLT, WMS-R, and WAIS-R administered as a battery to normals (Smith et al., 1992) and to dementia suspects (Smith et al., 1993). These five constructs were labeled Verbal Comprehension, Perceptual Organization, Attention/Concentration, Learning, and Retention. These labels were based on the measures that defined the factors and labels from prior factor analytic works with one or another of these instruments. Subsequently, Smith et al. (1994) demonstrated that a restricted subset of subtests from the WAIS-R, WMS-R, and AVLT could be used to accurately estimate the full factor scores for each of the above-named five factors. Identifying a reduced number of subtests provides an economy in the assessment of older persons with this battery. The scores derived from this shortened set of subtests were labeled the Mayo Cognitive Factors Scales (MCFS) and were normed to have a common mean (106) and standard deviation (12) to provide interfactor comparisons.

Comparing Cognitive Domains

An ensuing MOANS study (Ivnik et al., 1995) examined the degree of association between each of the five factors. Table 4–3 lists the intercorrelation of the factors among themselves at a single point in time. These data demonstrated that the degree of association between cognitive factors varies, even within a particular assessment. These findings challenged several long-held assumptions in neuropsychology. The first assumption was that an individual's level of cognitive function was relatively constant across cognitive domains. It has long been assumed that performance in one domain of cognitive function provides a reasonable estimate for performance in most other domains (Lezak, 1995). For example, it has been assumed that a person with a strong vocabulary should also have an excellent memory. When a person presents with above-average vocabulary skills and only average memory skills, that person is believed to have experienced a decline in memory. The Ivnik et al. (1995) data demonstrated that there is actually considerable variability in normal older adults across different skills, and that these differences negate the assumption of cognitive consistency across domains. It appears that it is entirely "normal" to display a statistically significant difference between two cognitive domains.

This study (Ivnik et al., 1995) also examined the stability of MCFS indices over a 1–2 year interval. The Pearson correlations between scores obtained from a MOANS sample over this interval for each of the five factors are listed in Table 4–4. These data helped to clarify that the stability of different cognitive factors

Table 4–3. Intercorrelations among Mayo Cognitive Factor Scale Scores

	VC	PO	AC	LRN	RET
VC	—	—	—	—	—
PO	.56	—	—	—	—
AC	.53	.47	—	—	—
LRN	.32	.37	.27	—	—
RET	.28	.38	.23	.47	—

Note: VC, Verbal Comprehension; PO, Perceptual Organization; AC, Attention/Concentration; LRN, Learning; RET, Retention.

Source: Ivnik et al. (1995).

Table 4–4. Stability Coefficients for Mayo Cognitive
Factor Scores of 1- to 2-Year Retest Intervals

Factor	Stability coefficient
Verbal Comprehension	.86
Perceptual Organization	.73
Attention/Concentration	.73
Learning	.69
Retention	.50

Source: Ivnik et al. (1995).

varies: differing cognitive domains have differing stabilities over time. This finding pointed to the need to "norm" longitudinal evaluations in order to better understand how much variability occurs in normal individuals across longitudinal assessment.

"Norming" Longitudinal Assessment

Longitudinal assessment of cognitive functioning is critical for studying the spectrum from normal aging to disease. Clinically, it can be difficult to distinguish disease-related cognitive change from normal cognitive change, even with the luxury of repeat cognitive assessment. This is because (*1*) some aspects of cognitive change are associated with normal aging; (*2*) some cognitive skills that are affected by normal aging are also affected by pathological conditions; and (*3*) cognitive change is insidious in most degenerative dementias. In the logical outgrowth of the previous stability study, Ivnik et al. (1999) examined group and individual change statistics in 93 cognitively-stable normals who had completed the MCFS battery on at least three occasions separated by roughly 1 year. In addition, 50 normal elderly, assessed four times over 5 years, were also studied.

Two unexpected findings emerged from this study. One finding involved practice effects—that is, the improvement in scores that is assumed to occur over successive administrations of the same tests. In the sample tested four times at 1- to 2-year intervals, practice effects were observed only between the first and second assessments. This finding was unexpected because repeated exposure to any test's content and procedures was assumed to enhance functioning over each repeat assessment, particularly for cognitively normal persons with good memories.

These data suggested otherwise: practice effects primarily influenced the results that are obtained at the first retesting. This is the same finding that Theisen et al. (1998) report in their study of selected WMS-R subtests that were readministered to normal people at much shorter (i.e., 2-week) test–retest intervals. By themselves, either of these studies' findings may be viewed with a degree of skepticism. However, when the same finding occurs in two entirely independent studies, it is difficult to dismiss. This finding calls into question prior assumptions about patterns of practice effects in longitudinal assessment.

A second finding was the rather large change-score sizes that are needed for test–retest changes to be considered pathologic. The data suggested that in order to have 90% confidence that an observed MCFS change score is abnormal (i.e., reflects true change), those scores must change on the order of 10 to 20 points without correcting for practice. When practice corrections are included, change scores still must range from 8 to 15 points, depending on the cognitive ability that is being examined. Table 4–5 lists the MCFS change scores necessary to have 90% confidence that a change has occurred that goes beyond normal test–retest variance.

Two factors contribute to the need for relatively large change scores to ensure that greater-than-normal change has occurred:

1. The standard error of a difference score is larger than the standard error associated with the individual scores from which it is derived.
2. Since confidence intervals (CI) for determining real change are based on the distribution of difference scores and these CI are frequently large; cognitive skills, when measured at reasonably global levels, differ widely in their stability over time.

Across the five general cognitive areas assessed by the MCFS, acquired verbal knowledge and verbal reasoning (i.e., MCFS-VC) are most stable over time. Nonverbal reasoning, attention, and concentration (i.e., PO and AC) are less stable, and the more dynamic abilities to learn and remember newly acquired information (i.e., LRN and RET) are least stable. This information has become available only as a result of longitudinal co-norming

Table 4–5. Inferring Real Change: 90% Confidence Intervals for MCFS Change Scores

MCFS score	Change score for 90% confidence deterioration has occurred	Change score for 90% confidence improvement has occurred
Verbal Comprehension (VC)	−8	+12
Perceptual Organization (PO)	−8	+19
Attention/Concentration (AC)	−12	+16
Learning (LRN)	−11	+24
Retention	−15	+25

Source: Adapted from Ivnik et al. (1995).

of tests. It is an ironic coincidence that these varying stabilities for cognitively normal people are inversely parallel to the relative sensitivities of different cognitive skills to the spectrum of conditions on the continuum from normal aging to common dementias.

It is important to stress that different cognitive abilities (as measured by the MCFS) require different magnitudes of change at identical confidence levels even though the normative groups' psychometric properties (i.e., means and standard deviations) for each measure are highly similar. In applied settings it has been common to assume that a person's cognitive abilities are stable (i.e., almost constant) over time and that most change reflects either measurement error or pathology. Since objective determinations of normal stability over clinically relevant time periods were not previously available, some investigators used a test's group-defined psychometric properties (e.g., standard deviation, standard error of measurement) to guide their thinking about change scores. But this practice incorrectly assumes that group variability in MCFS scores (or other standard scores) obtained at one time has implications for individual variability in the same scale's change scores over time. This practice does not recognize the fact that cognitive abilities possess differing degrees of temporal stability. Just as a person's physical capacities (e.g., blood pressure, vital capacity, strength) fluctuate over time and in response to numerous internal and external factors, it is both logical and reasonable to anticipate that cognitive skills also fluctuate over time and in response to many different biological, psychological, and environmental influences (e.g., fatigue, emotional status, medicines, and stress). Moreover, some cognitive skills are more prone to fluctuations than others. The Ivnik et al. (1999) data highlight that different cognitive abilities possess different degrees of temporal stability and that it may be incorrect to attribute all observed instability to either measurement error or pathology. There is no reason to assume that extraneous factors influence cognitive functioning in ways that are easily modeled by statistics. For example, such factors may not influence cognitive performance in a statistically linear manner.

GROUP VERSUS INDIVIDUAL STATISTICS: THE CLINICIAN'S PERSPECTIVE

Over the course of the MOANS studies, there has been an attempt to provide data in a format of greatest use to clinicians. Often, it is not the group summary statistics, such as means or Pearson r-values that have direct application for clinicians. For example, if a 75-year-old patient displays a 15-point split between the MCFS Learning and Verbal Comprehension scores, the knowledge that Learning and Verbal Comprehension correlate at the $r = .32$ level is of limited use. However, knowing that in a sample of normal older adults, 28% of the people have a discrepancy score of 15 points or greater between Verbal Comprehension and Learning informs clinical inference by revealing that such a discrepancy is relatively common in older adults. Similar frequency data from Ivnik et al. (1995) enables clinicians to determine that a change as small as 10 points in Verbal Comprehension was as rare in normal older adults as a change on the order of 25 points in Retention scores. While this follows from the relatively lower stability coefficient for Retention scores in normal samples, it is the frequency data (i.e., individual statistics) that translate the stability information into data that are directly relevant to clinical decision making.

In several other MOANS analyses, a similar attempt was made to supplement validation (group) statistics with individual statistics needed for clinical inference (e.g., Ivnik et al., 2001). For example, numerous researchers (Nelson and O'Connell, 1978; Crawford et al., 1988; Blair and Spreen, 1989; Brayne and

Beardsall, 1990; Grober and Sliwinski, 1991; Sharpe and O'Carroll, 1991; Johnstone and Wilhelm, 1996) have suggested that word recognition reading scores provide a means of estimating premorbid IQ in the face of early to moderate dementia. Using the longitudinal data from the MOANS sample, an attempt was made to validate this practice. Smith et al. (1997) identified a group of patients for whom IQ was established while they still met criteria for being "normal," but who displayed a decline in general cognitive functioning at longitudinal follow-up. This follow-up occurred, on average, 3.5 years after the normal IQ score was obtained. In these patients showing cognitive decline, word recognition scores obtained at follow-up were found to correlate at the $r = .70$ level with the verbal IQ scores obtained when the patients were still "normal." This correlation, a group statistic, provided evidence for the validity of the method of using word recognition scores to estimate premorbid IQ. It did not provide information on how to actually apply the technique clinically.

Typically, premorbid data is not available and the clinician is comparing a verbal IQ score with a contemporaneous word recognition reading score and inferring that a lower verbal IQ score, implies a decline in verbal IQ. However, how much lower does it need to be? To answer this question, individual statistics from normative neuropsychological data were needed. Smith et al. (1997) provided this clinically relevant data in the form of a frequency analysis in 271 normals. They calculated the frequency of various magnitudes of discrepancies between contemporaneous word recognition–based estimates of verbal IQ and actual verbal IQ. They were thus able to document that actual verbal IQ scores fall more than 9 points below estimated premorbid IQ in only 6% of a normal sample. This provides a cutoff score (>9 point discrepancy) that can be applied in the clinical evaluation of an individual.

Examining "hit rates," instead of group mean differences, is another example of emphasizing clinically relevant statistical approaches. In the clinical validation studies of the MCFS, null hypothesis testing revealed that all five MCFS scores displayed statistically significant mean differences when a normal sample was compared to a clinical sample comprised mostly of incident dementia cases (Ivnik et al., 1994). However, the means comparisons are group statistics. They were supplemented with logistic regression modeling. Logistic regression examines the adequacy of predictor variables in classifying cases. This technique can generate cut scores and classification accuracy statistics. In the MCFS validation study (Ivnik et al., 1994), logistic regression analysis suggested that the single index MCFS Retention was a good predictor of clinical status (optimal sensitivity/specificity = .72/.87). This single index was a better predictor than an index of interfactor variability. These findings implied that comparison of a single key cognitive index to within-group norms was clinically more useful than examination of within-subject interfactor variability. That is, absolute memory function relative to norms, as opposed to relative memory weakness based on within-subject comparisons, was a better predictor of clinical status. This argues against the hallowed practice in neuropsychology of comparing a person's cognitive scores to an estimated level of general function for that individual. This idiographic approach has been described as "indirect deficit measurement" (Lezak, 1995, p. 102). A nomothetic approach to direct deficit measurement using normative standards produces better hit rates. The nomothetic, direct deficit–measurement approach requires normative neuropsychological data (Lezak, 1995).

The longitudinal study of the MOANS cohort enabled us to attempt an additional study on the use of relative rather than absolute memory impairment in distinguishing among conditions along the spectrum from normal aging to disease. In a study by Malec and colleagues (1996), cluster analysis was used to establish "profiles" of Mayo Cognitive Factor Scores. Four profile types, three involving relative memory weakness, were selected a priori as likely to be associated with increased risk for the development of dementia. The cohort of normals on which the cluster analysis was based was followed for 3 to 4 years. Some 6% of this cohort developed cognitive impairment in this interval; this was twice the expected cumulative incidence expected for this period. Membership in one of the four at-risk clusters was associated with increased risk for development of cognitive impairment. Of the 16 persons who displayed cognitive impairment, 10 (63%) were from the at-risk clusters. Moreover, persons from the at-risk clusters were seven times more likely to display cognitive impairment at follow-up since 21% (10/47) of the members of the at-risk clusters developed cognitive impairment compared to just 3% (6/238) of the members of the non-risk clusters. However, considered from the individual case perspective, these numbers also reveal that at-risk profiles were "excessively sensitive." The analysis reveals that 37/47 (79%) of the at-risk members did not display cognitive decline in this interval. This analysis highlights the difference between sensitivity and positive predictive value. While almost two-thirds of the patients who developed cognitive impairment were captured by at-risk profiles, more than three-fourths of the members of the at-risk cohort did not go on to display cognitive impairment in this interval. This is possible because the overall base rate of incipient dementia was so low at 6% (in spite of being twice expectations from epidemiological studies). The low base rate, in contrast, enhanced the power of the non-risk profile, as a very strong indication that cognitive impairment would not develop in the interval. In other words, absence of the at-risk profile had substantial negative predictive value. Masur and colleagues (1994) had previously conducted a similar study and found that relative weakness on memory tests was a statistically significant predictor of which normals from the Bronx Aging study would convert to cognitive impairment during longitudinal follow-up. At comparable negative predictive values, their positive predictive value in that study was approximately two times greater than in the Malec et al. study (1996), but the cumulative incidence (i.e., base rate) was also over three times higher in the Masur et al. (1994) study.

Epidemiological Concepts and Neuropsychological Screening
Comparison of the Malec et al. (1996) and Mazur et al. (1994) analyses emphasizes the importance of distinguishing sensitivity and specificity from positive and negative predictive value. *Sensitivity* refers to the frequency with which members of a given group have a positive score on some criterion. In identification of dementia, for example, sensitivity is the percentage of a cohort of dementia patients who score below the cutoff on a memory test. *Specificity* refers to the frequency of negative scores on the criterion among persons without the target condition. Within the dementia example above, specificity refers to the percentage of time a cohort of normals score above a cutoff on a given memory task. In clinical practice, sensitivity and specificity statistics are

akin to group statistics. They are not very informative when interpreting the data from an individual because these data apply to groups of people with predetermined status. However, the clinician dealing with the spectrum from normal aging to dementia is confronted with people who are undiagnosed, not with people with defined conditions. In this situation, the clinically informative validation statistics are positive and negative predictive value.

The positive predictive value of a test refers to the probability that a person scoring below some cutoff on that test will display the target condition. Negative predictive value refers to the probability that a person scoring above the test cutoff will not display the condition. In other words, these statistics reflect the probability that a person with a given test score does or does not have the condition. Of course, positive and predictive negative value have mathematical associations with sensitivity and specificity. These associations are illustrated in Figure 4–2. More pragmatically, Table 4–6 depicts positive and negative predictive values as a function of the base rate of a condition and the sensitivity and specificity of a test. As can be inferred from the table, the positive and negative predictive probabilities are substantially influenced by the base rate of the condition in the individuals under study. One common error in the application of these statistics is to assume that prevalence of a condition in the general population is the relevant base rate in a given research study or clinical application. However, for patients being seen in a memory disorders clinic, for example, the base rate of dementia is not that of the general population. In fact, the base rate of dementia in memory clinics is probably exceedingly high. In these settings, the premium for the clinician may be on identifying conditions that do not reflect dementia but have some other

$$\text{Positive Predictive Value} = 100 * \frac{\text{Base Rate} * \text{Sensitivity}}{\text{Base Rate} * \text{Sensitivity} + (1 - \text{Base Rate}) * (1 - \text{Specificity})}$$

$$\text{Negative Predictive Value} = 100 * \frac{(1 - \text{Base Rate}) * \text{Specificity}}{(1 - \text{Base Rate}) * \text{Specificity} + \text{Base Rate} * (1 - \text{Sensitivity})}$$

Figure 4–2. Mathematical association of sensitivity, specificity, and positive and negative predictive value.

Table 4–6. Relationship of Positive and Negative Predictive Value to Base Rate, Sensitivity, and Specificity

Base rate	Sensitivity	Specificity	Positive predictive value (%)	Negative predictive value (%)
1/1000	0.90	0.90	0.89	99.99
	0.95	0.90	0.94	99.99
	0.90	0.95	1.77	99.99
	0.95	0.95	1.87	99.99
1/100	0.90	0.90	8.33	99.89
	0.95	0.90	8.76	99.94
	0.90	0.95	15.38	99.89
	0.95	0.95	16.10	99.95
1/10	0.90	0.90	50.00	98.97
	0.95	0.90	51.35	99.39
	0.90	0.95	66.67	98.84
	0.95	0.95	67.86	99.42

explanation. In other words, in these settings, negative predictive value may have equal or greater importance then positive predictive value.

Current studies of mild cognitive impairment do often focus on community- or population-based cohorts of older persons. In studies on the usefulness of neuropsychological measures in detection of MCI cases, the relevant base rate is still an important consideration. In these studies, MCI cases can be considered analogous to the epidemiological concept of an incident case. In other words, incidence rate may be the relevant base rate in such studies. Population-based studies at the Mayo Clinic (Kokmen et al., 1993) and elsewhere (Launer et al., 1999) have revealed annual incidence rates of 2.6% to 8.5%, even in persons over age 85. In studies where a much higher annual incidence rate occurs in the cohort, a bias in recruitment of "normals" may be operating. Table 4–5 suggests that overestimates of the base rate of the condition will result in overly optimistic positive predictive values.

Using Neuropsychological Norms in the Definition of MCI

As defined by Petersen in Chapter 1 in this volume, MCI persons are at elevated risk for developing dementia but are not universally early dementia cases. Thus, the identification of MCI cases might be conceptualized as a desire to identify persons with performances that have high positive predictive value for dementia. As can be seen in Table 4–6, slight increases in specificity have a more substantial effect on positive predictive value than slight increases of sensitivity. Age adjustments to neuropsychological scores reduces the likelihood of scoring below a cutoff score because of age-related variance, as opposed to disease-related variance. This is tantamount to increasing specificity, which, in turn, has a substantial effect on the positive predictive value of neuropsychological scores.

Conventional versus Robust Norms

As an aside, it should also be noted that the cutoff scores used in many studies do not reside within the tests. Clinicians can choose to adjust the cutoff score they select according to demographic parameters and epidemiological data. Sliwinski et al. (1996; see also Chapter 5 in this volume) have argued that use of age-adjusted norms in studies of older adults undermines the optimal sensitivity of measures because normative samples are often contaminated with preclinical cases. The relative importance of optimizing specificity versus sensitivity was discussed above. This issue notwithstanding, Sliwinski et al. (1996) report research showing that if one uses a score of -2 SDs or less as a cutoff, many cases of early dementia go undetected. The use of scores 2 SD below the mean for normals acknowledges the fact that any sample may contain a small number of abnormal cases. This is why one selects a cutoff score that is statistically rare for normals, but still within the parameters of a normal distribution. However, selecting -2 SDs as a rigid cutoff is not something clinicians are required to do. Receiver operating curves can still be used to identify ideal cutoffs for distinguishing between cohorts of dementia patients and cohorts of normal controls after age adjustments are made, and the cutoffs can be calculated for age-specific groups. If the base rate of the condition is relatively higher than the second percentile (i.e., the percentile associated with a score of -2 SDs), clinicians can choose to establish a higher cutoff score for identifying dementia cases. Of course the presence of large numbers of incipient dementia cases in a normative cohort will bias norms. However, the presence of this large number of cases suggests that the cohort is not an adequate representative of a normative sample. By definition, a normative sample should not have a higher cumulative incidence rate of dementia than is present in the general population. Whenever it is true that the normative cohort has a cumulative incidence of dementia that is equal to or less than that expected for the general population, the biasing of norms by the presence of incident dementia cases is minimal.

CONCLUSION

The MOANS studies were conducted with the goal of better understanding the psychometric properties of neuropsychological tools when used with older adults. This understanding was felt to be a necessary precursor to the use of neuropsychological tests in the early detection of dementia or other older-adult cognitive disorders. It is known that a variety of demographic factors produce variability on neuropsychological tests. This demographic variability can obscure detection of test variability attributable to incipient disease. The MOANS studies endeavored to better understand the contribution of these demographic factors in older adults and to provide adjustments for these. The focus was on provision of norms in a manner that is most useful to the clinician who is interpreting individual test scores. To this end, the MOANS studies have included procedures for norming common tests up until life's latest ages, co-norming IQ and memory measures, and using advanced statistical techniques to establish factor structure and hierarchical regression to identify the minimal number of subtests necessary to adequately measure these factors. Normative data were developed not just for use with initial neuropsychological evaluations but also for interpreting longitudinal data. The MOANS procedures appear to have influenced the new revisions of the Wechsler IQ and Memory scales, the WAIS-III and the Wechsler Memory Scale-III (The Psychological Corporation, 1997). The recognition that tests should be normed on persons over age 74 alone is a significant advancement. The adoption of other techniques also used in the MOANS studies reflects the effect that normative neuropsychological studies of older persons can have on the psychometric field in general. It is hoped that these normative neuropsychological procedures have improved the instrumentation used to assess normal older adults. Further, it is hoped that this helps more accurately place persons on the conceptual continuum from optimal aging to obvious dementia, including contributing to the recognition of mild cognitive impairment.

References

Albert, M. (1988). Cognitive function. In Geriatric Neuropsychology, edited by M. Albert and M. Moss (pp. 33–56). New York: Guilford Press.

Baltes, P., and H. Reese. (1984). The life span perspective in developmental psychology. In Developmental Psychology: An Advanced Textbook, edited by M. Bornstein and M. Lamb (pp. 493–532). Hillsdale, NJ: Erlbaum.

Blair, J., and O. Spreen. (1989). Predicting premorbid IQ: a revision of the National Adult Reading Test. *Clin Neuropsychol* 3:129–136.

Bolla, K., K. Lindgren, C. Bonaccorsy, and M. Bleecker. (1991). Memory complaints in older adults. *Arch Neurol* 48:61–64.

Brayne, C., and L. Beardsall. (1990). Estimation of verbal intelligence in an elderly community: an epidemiological study using the NART. *Br J Clin Psychol* 29:217–233.

Caine, E. (1993). Should aging-associated cognitive decline be included in DSM-IV? *J Neuropsychiatry Clin Neurosci* 5:1–5.

Crawford, J., J. Besson, and D. Parker. (1988). Estimation of pre-morbid intelligence in organic conditions. *Br J Psychiatry* 153:178–181.

Crook, T., R. Bartus, S. Ferris, P. Whitehouse, G. Cohen, and S. Gershon (1986). Age-associated memory impairment: proposed diagnostic criteria and measures of clinical change—Report of a National Institute of Mental Health Work Group. *Devel Neuropsychol* 2:261–276.

Grober, E., and M. Sliwinski. (1991). Development and validation of a model for estimating premorbid verbal intelligence in the elderly. *J Clin Exper Neuropsychol* 13:933–949.

Hanninen, T., K. Reinikainen, E.-L. Helkala, K. Koivisto, L. Mykkanen, M. Laakso, K. Pyorala, and P. Riekkinen. (1994). Subjective memory complaints and personality traits in normal elderly subjects. *J Am Geriatr Soc* 42(1):1–4.

Ivnik, R., J. Malec, G. Smith, and E. Tangalos. (1992a). Mayo's Older Americans Normative Studies: WAIS-R norms for ages 56–97. *Clin Neuropsychol* 6(Suppl):1–30.

Ivnik, R., J. Malec, G. Smith, and E. Tangalos. (1992b). Mayo's Older Americans Normative Studies: WAIS-R, WMS-R and AVLT norms for ages 56–97. *Clin Neuropsychol* 6(Suppl):1–104.

Ivnik, R., J. Malec, G. Smith, E. Tangalos, and R. Petersen. (1996). Neuropsychological tests' norms above age 55: COWAT, BNT, MAE Token, WRAT-R reading, AMNART, STROOP, TMT, and JLO. *Clin Neuropsychol* 10:262–278.

Ivnik, R.J., G.E. Smith, J. Cerhan, B.F. Boeve, E.G. Tangalos, and R.C. Petersen. (2001). Understanding cognitive tests' diagnostic capabilities. *Clin Neuropsychol* 15(1):114–124.

Ivnik, R.J., G.E. Smith, J.A. Lucas, R.C. Petersen, B.F. Boeve, E. Kokmen, and E.G. Tangalos. (1999). Testing normal older people three or four times at 1- to 2-year intervals: defining normal variance. *Neuropsychology* 13:121–127.

Ivnik, R., G. Smith, J. Malec, R. Petersen, E. Kokmen, and E. Tangalos. (1994). MOANS Cognitive Factor Scales (MCFS): distinguishing normal and clinical samples by profile variability. *Neuropsychology* 8:203–209.

Ivnik, R., G. Smith, J. Malec, R. Petersen, and E. Tangalos. (1995). Long-term stability and inter-correlations of cognitive abilities in older persons. *Psychol Assess J Consulting Clin Psychol* 7:155–161.

Johnstone, B., and K. Wilhelm. (1996). The longitudinal stability of the WRAT-R Reading subtest: is it an appropriate estimate of premorbid intelligence? *J Int Neuropsychol Soc* 2:282–285.

Kahn, R., S. Zarit, N. Hilbert, and G. Niederehe. (1975). Memory complaint and impairment in the aged: the effect of depression and altered brain function. *Arch General Psychiatry* 32:1569–1573.

Kokmen, E., C. Beard, P. O'Brien, K. Offord, and L. Kurland. (1993). Is the incidence of dementing illness changing? A 25-year time trend study in Rochester, Minnesota (1960–1984). *Neurology* 43:1887–1892.

Larrabee, G., and H. Levin. (1986). Memory self-ratings and objective test performance in a normal elderly sample. *J Clin Exp Neuropsychol* 8:275–284.

LaRue, A. (1992). Aging and Neuropsychological Assessment. New York: Plenum Press.

Launer, L., K. Andersen, M. Dewey, L. Letenneur, A. Ott, L. Amaducci, C. Brayne, J. Copeland, J. Dartigues, P. Kragh-Sorensen, A. Lobo, J. Martinez-Lage, T. Stijnen, and A. Hofman. (1999). Rates and risk factors for dementia and Alzheimer's disease: results from EURODEM pooled analyses. *Neurology* 52(1):78–84.

Lezak, M. (1995). Neuropsychological Assessment, 3rd ed. New York: Oxford University Press.

Lucas, J., R. Ivnik, G. Smith, D. Bohac, E. Tangalos, N. Graff-Radford, and R. Petersen. (1998a). Mayo older American studies: category fluency norms. *J Clin Exp Neuropsychol* 20:194–200.

Lucas, J., R. Ivnik, G. Smith, D. Bohac, E. Tangalos, E. Kokmen, N. Graff-Radford, and R. Petersen. (1998b). Normative data for the Mattis Dementia Rating Scale. *J Clin Exp Neuropsychol* 20:536–547.

Malec, J., R. Ivnik, and G. Smith. (1993). Neuropsychology and normal aging: clinicians' perspective. In Neuropsychology of Alzheimer's Disease and Related Dementias, edited by R. Parks, R. Zec, and R. Wilson (pp. 81–111). New York: Oxford University Press.

Malec, J., G. Smith, R. Ivnik, R. Petersen, and E. Tangalos. (1996). Clusters of "impaired" normal elderly do not decline cognitively in 3–5 years. *Neuropsychology* 10:66–73.

Masur, D., M. Sliwinski, R. Lipton, A. Blau, and H. Crystal. (1994). Neuropsychological prediction of dementia and the absence of dementia in healthy elderly persons. *Neurology* 44:1427–1432.

McGlone, J., S. Gupta, D. Humphrey, S. Oppenheimer, T. Mirsen, and D. Evans. (1990). Screening for early dementia using memory complaints from patients and relatives. *Arch Neurol* 47:1189–1193.

McKhann, G., D. Drachman, M. Folstein, R. Katzman, D. Price, and E. Stadlan. (1984). Clinical diagnosis of Alzheimer's disease: report of the NINCDS-ADRDA work group under the auspices of Department of Health and Human Services task force on Alzheimer's disease. *Neurology* 34:939–944.

Monsch, A., M. Bondi, N. Butters, J. Paulsen, D. Salmon, P. Brugger, and M. Swenson. (1994). A comparison of category and letter fluency in Alzheimer's disease and Huntington's disease. *Neuropsychology* 8(1):25–30.

Nelson, H., and A. O'Connell. (1978). Dementia: the estimation of premorbid intelligence levels using the New Adult Reading Test. *Cortex* 14: 234–244.

O'Connor, D., A. Pollitt, M. Roth, P. Brook, and B. Reiss. (1989). Memory complaints and impairment in normal, depressed, and demented elderly persons identified in a community survey. *Arch Gerontol Geriatr* 1(Suppl):151–163.

Pauker, J. (1988). Constructing overlapping cell tables to maximize the clinical usefulness of normative test data: rationale and an example from neuropsychology. *J Clin Psychol* 44:930–933.

Petersen, R.C. (2003). Conceptual overview. In Mild Cognitive Impairment: Aging to Alzheimer's Disease, edited by R.C. Petersen (pp. 1–14). New York: Oxford University Press.

Petersen, R., G. Smith, E. Kokmen, R. Ivnik, and E. Tangalos. (1992). Memory function in normal aging. *Neurology* 42:396–401.

Petersen, R., G. Smith, R. Ivnik, E. Kokmen, and E. Tangalos. (1994). Memory function in very early Alzheimer's disease. *Neurology* 44:867–872.

Plotkin, D., J. Mintz, and L. Jarvik. (1985). Subjective memory complaints in geriatric depression. *Am J Psychiatry* 142:1103–1105.

Powell, D. (1994). Profiles in Cognitive Aging. Cambridge, MA: Harvard University Press.

The Psychological Corporation. (1997). WAIS-III-WMS-III: Technical Manual. San Antonio, TX: The Psychological Corporation.

Rey, A. (1964). L'examen clinique en psychologie. Paris: Presses Universitaires de France.

Rowe, J., and R. Kahn. (1987). Human aging: usual and successful. *Science* 237:143–149.

Schroots, J., and J. Birren. (1996). History, concepts, and theory in the psychology of aging. In Handbook of the Psychology of Aging, edited by J. Birren and K. Schaie, 4th ed. (pp. 3–23). San Diego: Academic Press.

Sharpe, K., and R. O'Carroll. (1991). Estimating premorbid intellectual level in dementia using the National Adult Reading Test: a Canadian study. *Br J Clin Psychol* 30:381–384.

Sliwinski, et al. Use of normative neuropsychological data. In Aging and Mild Cognitive Impairment, edited by R.C. Petersen. New York: Oxford University Press.

Sliwinski, M., R. Lipton, H. Buschke, and W. Stewart. (1996). The effects of preclinical dementia on estimates of normal cognitive function in aging. *J Gerontol Psychol Sci* 51(B):217–225.

Smith, G., R. Ivnik, R. Petersen, J. Malec, E. Kokmen, and E. Tangalos. (1991). Age-associated memory impairment diagnoses: problems of reliability and concerns for terminology. *Psychol Aging* 6:551–558.

Smith, G., R. Ivnik, J. Malec, R. Petersen, E. Tangalos, and L. Kurland. (1992). Mayo's Older Americans Normative Studies (MOANS): factor structure of a core battery. *Psychol Assess J Consulting Clin Psychol* 4:382–390.

Smith, G., R. Ivnik, J. Malec, and E. Tangalos. (1993). Factor structure of the MOANS core battery: replication in a clinical sample. *Psychol Assess J Consulting Clin Psychol* 5:121–124.

Smith, G., R. Petersen, R. Ivnik, J. Malec, and E. Tangalos. (1996). Subjective memory complaints, psychological distress, and longitudinal change in objective memory performance. *Psychol Aging* 11:272–279.

Smith, G., D. Bohac, R. Ivnik, and J. Malec. (1997). Using word recognition tests to estimate premorbid IQ in early dementia patients: longitudinal data. *J Int Neuropsycholog Soc* 3:528–533.

Smith, G.E., R.J. Ivnik, J.F. Malec, R.C. Petersen, E. Kokmen, and E.G. Tangalos. (1994). Mayo and cognitive factor scales: derivation of a short battery and norms for factor scores. *Neuropsychology* 8:194–202.

Smith, G., E. Kokmen, and P. O'Brien. (2000). Risk factors for nursing home placement in a population-based dementia cohort. *J Am Geriatr Soc* 48:519–525.

Taylor, J., T. Miller, and J. Tinklenberg. (1992). Correlates of memory decline: a 4-year longitudinal study of older adults with memory complaints. *Psychol Aging* 7:185–193.

Theisen, M.E., L.J. Rapport, B.N. Axelrod, and D.B. Brines. (1998). Effects of practice in repeated administrations of the Weschler Memory Scale-Revised in normal adults. *Assessment* 5:85–92.

Wechsler, D. (1981). Wechsler Adult Intelligence Scale–Revised. New York: Psychological Corporation.

Wechsler, D. (1987). Wechsler Memory Scale–Revised. New York: Psychological Corporation.

Welsh, K., N. Butters, J. Hughes, R. Mohs, and A. Heyman. (1991). Detection of abnormal memory decline in mild cases of Alzheimer's disease using CERAD neuropsychological measures. *Arch Neurol* 48:278–281.

CHAPTER **5**

Optimizing Cognitive Test Norms
for Detection

MARTIN SLIWINSKI
RICHARD LIPTON
HERMAN BUSCHKE
CHRISTINA WASYLYSHYN

Neuropsychological testing is often used to provide objective and sensitive evidence of mild cognitive impairment in older adults that may indicate the presence of a dementing illness such as Alzheimer's disease (AD). Unfortunately, standard techniques for norming cognitive tests in older adults can diminish a test's discriminative validity for detecting mild cognitive impairment caused by the early stages of Alzheimer's disease. The focus of this chapter is on how to construct norms that are optimal for detecting mild cognitive impairment caused by preclinical Alzheimer's disease (pAD).

Traditional methods for norming psychological tests involve statistically correcting for age differences. Although they are useful for comparative purposes, age-correcting cognitive test scores can significantly diminish test sensitivity for detecting mild cognitive impairment caused by AD. The reason that traditional techniques for norming diminish test sensitivity is that they rely on statistical methods that model performance on cognitive tests as a function of age, but they do not consider how either age or test performance relates to the likelihood of having pAD. Our contention is that norms, if they are to be used for detecting mild cognitive impairment, should rely on statistical methods that directly model the probability of having pAD as a function of test performance and age. This subtle, but critically important, distinction will become clearer as we consider two approaches to norming cognitive tests in older adult populations and evaluate their appropriateness for detecting pAD.

First, we reframe the problem of detecting mild cognitive impairment to one of detecting preclinical dementia (i.e., preclinical Alzheimer's disease, or pAD). We define pAD as that stage in the disease during which pathological changes in the brain have begun to affect cognition, but in which impairment is too mild to meet established criteria for AD or to cause functional problems (Reifler, 1997). Second, we discuss the epidemiology of Alzheimer's disease and its implications for developing optimal norms for the detection of cognitive impairment in older adults. Third, we contrast two types of norms—comparative and diagnostic—and the different types of questions they are useful (and not useful) for answering. Fourth, we consider practical issues of how to apply norms in various clinical and research settings. We conclude with a discussion of the relationship between cognitive aging and mild cognitive impairment: that is, are they part of the same continuum, or do they differ qualitatively?

MILD COGNITIVE IMPAIRMENT AND PRECLINICAL ALZHEIMER'S DISEASE

The term *mild cognitive impairment* has become almost synonymous with a specific classification scheme (Smith et al., 1996) and is referred to as *MCI*. While most researchers agree that MCI is a diagnostic entity, whose clinical diagnosis should be based on both structured clinical ratings and neuropsychological tests, there is debate about what to classify it as: a transitional state between normal aging and AD (Petersen, 2000), a subthreshold disorder (Reischies and Hellweg, 2000), a disease, or a combination of some or all of these categories. Our view is that MCI is a label assigned to individuals who are deemed to be at high risk for developing clinically diagnosable dementia. Regardless of how to interpret MCI, the key to its detection is defining memory impairment, as most of the patient's other cognitive functions are preserved. The remainder of this chapter is focused on how to improve the detection of cognitive impairment caused by an underlying disease process (e.g., AD) in older adults.

The arguments to be developed in this chapter rest on the following premise: cognitive impairment in older adults is caused by a disease process. And the most important and prevalent cause of cognitive impairment in older adults is AD. Thus, the problem of identifying mild cognitive impairment in older adults is really one of detecting preclinical dementia—in particular, pAD. This implies that candidate detection methods should be informed by the epidemiology of AD. Norms should provide information about the likelihood, or probability, that an individual has mild cognitive impairment caused by pAD, given a certain score on a cognitive test and other risk factors, such as a person's age.

Two types of information are needed to determine the probability of mild cognitive impairment caused by pAD, given a certain cognitive test score. The first is discriminative validity of the cognitive test. The discriminative validity of a test is appropriately conveyed by its sensitivity and specificity for detecting mild cognitive impairment. And to calculate sensitivity and specificity, information regarding the performance of the to-be-detected group must be used; normative information on the intact (unimpaired) group is not sufficient to determine discriminative validity. The second type of information is the base rate or prevalence of pAD, which can vary as a function of setting (e.g., outpatient clinic, community, nursing homes) and of person characteristics, such as age. For example, there is an increase in the prevalence of dementia from community dwelling to hospitalized to institutionalized patients, and this prevalence rises with age (Sui, 1991). Without these two types of information, the probability or likelihood that a person has mild cognitive impairment given a score on a cognitive test cannot be determined.

Although it is widely acknowledged that prevalence has a substantial influence on the chances of clinical AD for a given test score, norms rarely take explicit account of how base rate affects interpretation of test scores (Meiran et al., 1996). More relevant to the present discussion is the fact that (besides providing turnover rates), attempts at defining mild cognitive impairment (e.g., Petersen, 2000) offer no information about the expected prevalence of mild cognitive impairment or how it should affect clinical judgment. Also of concern is the practice of age-correcting test norms in order to infer cognitive impairment. This sort of correction will rarely be helpful and can diminish test sensitivity for detecting mild cognitive impairment caused by pAD, especially when the norms are applied outside of the sample used to develop them.

We now examine how a person's age affects the probability that he or she has pAD.

Considerable epidemiological research has shown a strong positive relationship between age and the prevalence of clinical AD (Katzman and Kawas, 1994). Similarly, and as expected, there is also a strong positive relationship between age and the probability of having pAD. We use data from the Einstein Aging Study (EAS), a longitudinal study of cognitive aging and dementia, to illustrate this relationship. Figure 5–1 shows the relationship between age at baseline and the probability of developing clinically diagnosable AD within 5 years. None of the individuals who con-

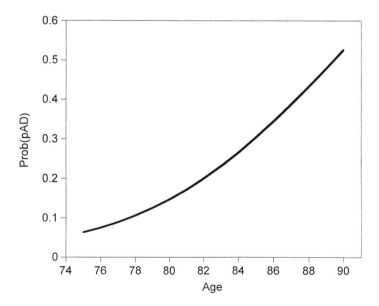

Figure 5–1. Probability of developing clinically diagnosable Alzheimer's disease within 5 years, by age. Data from the Einstein Aging Study [Sliwinski et al. (1997)].

tributed data to this analysis met established diagnostic criteria for dementia or made more than eight errors on the Blessed Information, Memory and Concentration test at their baseline assessment (Blessed et al., 1968). We defined as having pAD at baseline all persons who developed clinically diagnosable AD within 5 years of baseline testing. The prevalence of pAD increases with age because older persons are at greater risk for developing clinical AD.

The data shown in Figure 5–1 indicate that the older a person is, the more likely he or she is to have pAD. Consequently, the older a person is, the more likely he or she is to have mild cognitive impairment caused by pAD. The challenge facing diagnosticians is to detect the mild cognitive impairment caused by the very early stages of AD, before the disease has caused widespread cognitive impairment that results in functional decline.

We next examine how two methods of norming cognitive tests assist diagnosticians in making inferences regarding the likelihood of cognitive impairment given a test score. One method, comparative norming, models the relationship between age and test performance. The second method, diagnostic norming, directly models the relationship between the probability of having pAD and test performance. After describing these two methods, we will consider how the information provided by each can be used to infer and detect mild cognitive impairment in older adults.

COMPARATIVE AND DIAGNOSTIC TEST NORMS

Comparative norms are used to assess the relative rank of an individual with respect to a group of similar individuals. *Diagnostic norms* are used to discriminate individuals in two or more clinically defined groups, such as demented and nondemented older adults (Meiran et al., 1996; Sliwinski et al., 1997). Both types of norms make use of external information that, in the case of comparative norms, can affect performance on cognitive tests or, in the case of diagnostic norms, can affect the probability of AD. The most critical variable that affects both cognitive test scores and the probability of AD in older adults is a person's age. Older persons, on average, score lower on cognitive tests and are at increased risk for developing AD.

Now we will consider the nature of information provided by each type of norm and how each type of norm makes use of information about a person's age.

Comparative Norms

Comparative norms provide information in the form of means and standard deviations, or empirically estimated percentiles, that permit individuals to be judged relative to their age peers. These norms "correct" test scores by removing the effect of age so that the average test score across persons of different ages will be invariant. Statistically, this correction is accomplished by estimating the average score for a given age (either through ordinary least-squares regression or by computing mean scores separately for age strata), and then subtracting the age-specific mean from each person's test score.

To make the specifics of age correction more concrete, we present an example from published norms for the Selective Reminding Test (Buschke, 1973). These data were collected as part of the EAS (Sliwinski et al., 1997). The solid line in Figure 5–2 shows the average score on the Selective Reminding Test (sum of total recall) as a function of age in persons between the ages of 74 and 90. The regression coefficient of relating the average selective reminding score to age is $-.64$, which means that a 10-year difference in age corresponds to approximately a 6-point difference in the average sum score ($-.64 \times 10 = 6.4$). This regression indicates the average memory score is about 44 for 75-year-olds, 41 for 80-year-olds, and 38 for 85-year-olds. Now, assume that a 75-year-old (represented by the circle in Figure 5–2) and an 85-year-old (represented by the square in Figure 5–2) both score 30 on the test. Because the standard deviation is approximately 8, the age-corrected score for the 75-year-old is -1.75 standard units and the age-corrected score for the 85-year-old is -1.0 standard units. Thus, the same raw score (30) corresponds to the fourth percentile for the 75-year-old and to the sixteenth percentile for the 85-year-old.

How does one infer cognitive impairment based on age-corrected test scores? The inference is indirect and statistically uninformed, because age-corrected norms provide no informa-

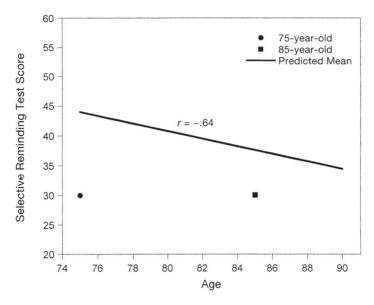

Figure 5–2. Absolute memory performance relative to predicted performance on the Selective Reminding Test (Buschke, 1973) as a function of age. Data from the Einstein Aging Study [Sliwinski et al. (1997)].

tion about discriminative validity or about how to incorporate prevalence information. One definition of mild cognitive impairment that relies on objective cognitive testing requires that individuals perform at least 1.5 SDs below the age-corrected mean on a test of memory (Petersen et al., 1995; Smith et al., 1996; Petersen et al., 1999; Reischies and Hellweg, 2000). Using this definition, we would identify the 75-year-old in the preceding example as having mild cognitive impairment because that person's score fell below 1.5 SDs from the age-appropriate mean. The 85-year-old would not be identified as impaired because that person's score fell within 1.5 SDs of the age-appropriate mean.

To be identified as impaired based on the Selective Reminding norms, a 75-year-old would need to score 32 or less, and an 85-year-old would need to score 26 or less. In this respect, impairment cut scores based on age-corrected comparative norms are *age-lenient*: that is, increasingly lower scores are needed to detect impairment in older individuals. We must point out that using age-corrected comparative norms to define mild cognitive impairment has demonstrated predictive validity, in that persons meeting this criterion are at a substantially higher risk for developing AD (Smith et al., 1996; Petersen et al., 1999). For example, individuals with MCI appear to be at a higher risk of developing AD at a rate of 12% to 15% per year (Kantarci et al., 2000). However, it is important to understand inherent limitations to this approach that compromise both its construct and predictive validity.

An important and undesirable consequence of age correcting is that the same proportion of the population will fall below *any* impairment cut score for all ages. By defining cognitive impairment with age-corrected test scores, one must assume that the prevalence of the entity to be detected does not vary as a function of age. Since we know that the prevalence of pAD increases as a function of age, one must question whether defining mild cognitive impairment as deviant age-corrected performance is an optimal method for identifying pAD. Consequently, we contend that both the construct and predictive validity of existing frameworks for defining mild cognitive in older adults can be improved by using norming methods that

1. Accurately reflect age-specific prevalence of pAD
2. Provide direct information of how a given score translates to the probability of impairment
3. Optimize the discrimination of intact and impaired individuals

We now consider such an alternative method for detecting mild cognitive impairment caused by pAD.

Diagnostic Norms

Diagnostic norms provide information in the form of cut scores, or probabilities, that can be used to classify individuals into one or more diagnostic groups. Comparative norms make use of only two pieces of information: the performance of intact persons on a cognitive test, and the relationship between age and test performance. Additional information is required to compute the probability that an individual has pAD. How the group to be detected (i.e., pAD) performs on the test and on age-specific and setting-specific (e.g., inpatient clinic, community, nursing home) prevalence rates of pAD are also needed to estimate the probability of pAD for any individual. Table 5–1 summarizes the type of information used by comparative and diagnostic norms.

Diagnostic norms are based on statistical methods (e.g., logistic regression) that make use of Baye's theorem to assign probabilities associated with a diagnostic outcome (for examples, see Elwood, 1993; Meiran et al., 1996; Buschke et al., 1997, 1999). First, we show how diagnostic norms are used to infer impairment in full-blown clinical AD. Then, we consider implications for using diagnostic norms to identify mild cognitive impairment caused by pAD.

The first step in constructing diagnostic norms for a cognitive test is to compute sensitivity and specificity for all possible cut scores. The trade-off between sensitivity and specificity is commonly displayed by the receiver operating characteristic (ROC) plot. Then, after specifying the sensitivity–specificity trade-off, one can compute the probability of impairment, given a test score for difference prevalence rates. An excellent example of this type of diagnostic norming is provided by Meiran et al. (1996). They provide tables that translate different scores on mental status tests into probabilities of having AD for different AD prevalence rates. For example, they report that a score of 25 on the Mini-Mental State Examination (MMSE) in community-residing adults between the ages of 65 and 74 corresponds to a .11 probability of AD. The same score for an older person (74 to 85) corresponds to a much higher probability of AD, .61. Thus, diagnostic norms provide age-weighted (in contrast to age-corrected) test scores so that age-specific prevalence rates are correctly incorporated into impairment probabilities.

Table 5–1. Information Used by Comparative and Diagnostic Norms

	TYPE OF NORM	
	Comparative	Diagnostic
Control test performance	X	X
pAD test performance		X
Test–age relationship	X	X
Age–pAD relationship		X
pAD baserate		X

X = present.

When age-specific increases in the prevalence of AD are properly incorporated into diagnostic decisions, the relative probability of impairment for a given test score may *increase* as age increases. In contrast, we demonstrated here that the likelihood of impairment inferred from age-corrected comparative norms must remain constant even as age increases. We addressed the effect of incorrectly correcting for age on diagnostic accuracy of the Selective Reminding Test (Sliwinski et al., 1997). We showed that, holding specificity constant, the sensitivity of age-corrected scores was about 25% lower than the sensitivity of age-weighted scores (52% vs. 78%, respectively). Thus, improper correction for age can significantly diminish test discriminative validity for detecting AD-related cognitive impairment.

Since AD and pAD share a similar age–risk relationship, we also expect age-correction to diminish test discriminative validity for detecting mild cognitive impairment. To address this issue, we examined the discriminative validity of two cognitive measures (selective reminding and category fluency) for detecting pAD in one of our EAS cohorts after the measures had been normed by age correction (i.e., comparative norming) or by age weighting (i.e., diagnostic norming).

Figures 5–3 and 5–4 show the ROC curves for the Selective Reminding Test and the Category Fluency Test, respectively. The dashed line in each figure shows the sensitivity–specificity trade-off for each measure after it had been corrected for age (i.e., age-corrected test scores were used). The solid line shows the sensitivity–specificity trade-off for test scores that were weighted for the age-specific prevalence rates of pAD in this sample. For both tests, the solid line falls above the dashed line, indicating higher sensitivities for detecting pAD for fixed values of specificity. The ROC analysis indicates that the discriminative validity of age-weighted test scores for detecting mild cognitive impairment caused by pAD is greater than the discriminative validity of age-corrected test scores.

INFERRING IMPAIRMENT WITH COMPARATIVE AND DIAGNOSTIC NORMS

Because the average memory score declines as a function of age, a given (raw) memory score indicates relatively better perfor-

Selective Reminding

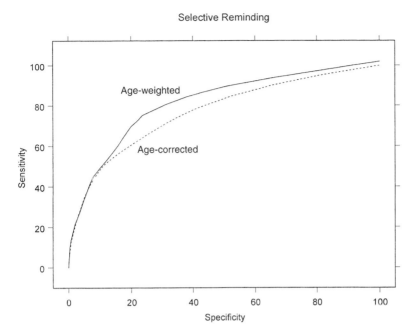

Figure 5–3. Receiver operating characteristic curves for age-corrected versus age-weighted scores on selective reminding.

mance for an older person than for a younger person. Thus, the logic behind age-corrected norms allows neuropsychologists to answer questions such as, "Given a person's age, is he or she performing above average, below average, or as expected?" This interpretation of age-corrected performance is intuitive and correct.

Does it also follow that the lower age-corrected scores are associated with an increased likelihood of cognitive impairment? Not necessarily. Specifically, it does *not* follow that a 75-year old who scores in the fourth percentile is more likely to have cognitive impairment than an 85-year-old who scores, for example, in the sixteenth percentile. Such inference requires information about the prevalence of cognitive impairment in general, how prevalence varies with age, and the discriminative validity of the specific test—none of which is conveyed by comparative norms. Because the prevalence of pAD increases with age, the probability of pAD for a given test score should be *higher* for older persons. Impairment inferences based on age-corrected comparative

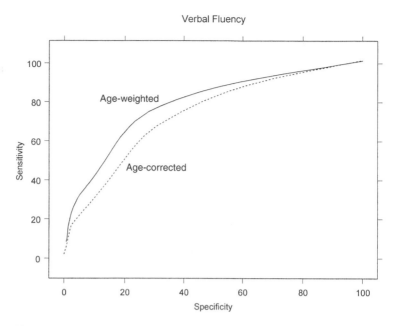

Figure 5–4. Receiver operating characteristic curves for age-corrected versus age-weighted scores on verbal fluency.

norms assume the opposite—namely, that the probability of impairment for a given test score will be *lower* for older persons.

Age-corrected comparative norms are not well suited to answer questions like "Given a person's memory score and age, what is the likelihood he or she has pAD?" Definitions of mild cognitive impairment as performance below an age-corrected cut score have poor construct validity if the construct to be measured is pAD. Such definitions have poor construct validity because they do not share a central epidemiological characteristic of pAD: namely, a positive association between risk of impairment and age. Although such definitions have demonstrated predictive validity, we contend, and have shown data to indicate, that predictive validity will be greater when diagnostic norms are used to infer mild cognitive impairment.

ARE COGNITIVE AGING AND MILD COGNITIVE IMPAIRMENT THE SAME?

We are not asserting that cognitive impairment in older adults caused by diseases other than AD (e.g., Lewy body disease, vascular disease) are in any way unimportant. Our position is that focusing on AD is important because it is so prevalent among older adults and because it is now a treatable disorder. In addition, by specifying the disease to be detected, one can more clearly define disease characteristics (e.g., risk factors and prevalence rates) and specify how that information should be used to construct optimal norms for detecting mild cognitive impairment.

By reframing the problem of identifying mild cognitive impairment into one of detecting pAD, we raise the question of whether age-related cognitive change (i.e., cognitive aging) differs from AD-related cognitive impairment only in severity or in kind. We will focus on memory because this cognitive domain is strongly affected by both age and AD. Memory declines in older adults with and without pAD can be placed on the same measurement continuum by virtue of using a common metric (i.e., performance on a memory test or tests). In this regard, one can correctly assert that memory impairment caused by pAD is more severe than the memory declines that accompany healthy aging. However, this does not imply that the memory changes seen in healthy aging and those caused by pAD differ *only* in severity.

Research from the EAS has provided evidence indicating that the memory impairment in AD differs not only in severity but also in kind from age-related memory changes. By using controlled learning procedures (Grober and Buschke, 1987) that control for attentional deficits, inefficient strategy use, and production deficits, many of the memory problems seen in healthy older adults can be ameliorated (Buschke and Grober, 1986; Grober and Buschke, 1987). In contrast, large memory deficits remain, and are sometimes exacerbated (Buschke et al., 1997), in demented older adults under conditions of controlled learning. This research suggests that the memory problems common in healthy older adults may be secondary to deficits in supportive cognitive functions, such as attention.

In fact, a growing body of research (see Salthouse, 1996, for a review) suggests that age-related memory differences may be a result of inefficient information processing that is caused by generalized cognitive slowing. In a recent study (Sliwinski and Buschke, 1997), we contrasted the role of processing speed as a mediator of age-related and dementia-related difference in cued recall and test memory. Consistent with previous research, statistical control of processing speed significantly attenuated or eliminated age differences on each of the memory measures. In contrast to the results for age differences, statistical control of processing speed did not significantly attenuate dementia-related memory deficits, suggesting that processing speed is not an important mediator of dementia-related memory impairment. Memory decline in healthy aging may be "secondary" to general declines in processing speed and efficiency, but memory impairment in dementia is "primary" in the sense that it is not mediated by a more general functional deficit. The results from Sliwinski and Buschke (1997) also suggest that memory impairment in dementia does not represent only a worsening of the memory decline that accompanies healthy aging, since if it did, one might reasonably expect that the same functional mechanisms (e.g., processing speed) should mediate cognitive impairment attributable to either aging or dementia.

CONCLUSIONS AND SUMMARY

Quite apart from the important theoretical issue of whether mild cognitive impairment (i.e., pAD) and healthy cognitive aging differ qualitatively or only quantitatively is a practical question: What kind of test norming should be done to provide optimal information for detecting pAD? Both comparative and diagnostic norms provide information that can be used for assigning individuals into high- and low-risk groups because poor memory performance is associated with dementia risk. However, only diagnostic tests provide direct information about how to translate a person's memory score and their age into a probability regarding their having mild cognitive impairment caused by pAD. Therefore, using diagnostic norms can improve the predictive validity of MCI classifications. Using diagnostic norms will also improve the construct validity of MCI. As currently defined, the rate of MCI is expected to be age invariant, a property that contradicts a well-established characteristic of dementia. Being classified as MCI should not result from having a low memory score relative to an individual's age peers, but from having a memory score that places an individual at a specifiable increased risk of developing clinical dementia. Only by relying on information provided by diagnostic norms can definition of mild cognitive impairment be brought into line with the underlying disease they are intended to indicate.

References

Blessed, G., B.E. Tomlinson, and M. Roth. (1968). The association between quantitative measures of dementia and of senile changes in the cerebral grey matter of elderly subjects. *British Journal of Psychiatry*, 114:797–811.

Buschke, H. (1973). Selective reminding for analysis of memory and learning. *J Verbal Learning Verbal Behav* 12:543–550.

Buschke, H. (1987).

Buschke, H., and E. Grober. (1986). Genuine memory deficits in age-associated memory impairment. *Devel Neuropsychol* 2:287–307.

Buschke, H., M. Sliwinski, G. Kuslansky, and R. Lipton. (1997). Diagnosis of early dementia by the Double Memory Test: encoding specificity improves diagnostic sensitivity and specificity. *Neurology* 48:989–997.

Buschke, H., G. Kuslansky, M. Katz, W.F. Stewart, M.J. Sliwinski, H.M. Eckholdt, and R.B. Lipton. (1999). Screening for dementia with the Memory Impairment Screen. *Neurology* 52:231–238.

Elwood, R.W. (1993). Clinical discriminations and neuropsychological tests: an appeal Bayes' Theorem. *Clin Neuropsychol* 7:224–233.

Grober, E., and H. Buschke. (1987). Genuine memory deficits in dementia. *Devel Neuropsychol* 3:13–36.

Kantarci, K., C.R. Jack Jr., Y.C. Xu, N.G. Campeau, P.C. O'Brien, G.E. Smith, R.J. Ivnik, B.F. Boeve, E. Kokmen, E.G. Tangalos, and R.C. Petersen. (2000). Regional metabolic patterns in mild cognitive impairment and Alzheimer's disease: a ^{1}H MRS study. *Neurology* 55:210–217.

Katzman, R., and C. Kawas. (1994). The epidemiology of dementia and Alzheimer's disease. In Alzheimer's Disease, edited by R. Katzman, R.D. Terry, and K.L. Bick (pp. 105–122). New York: Raven Press.

Meiran N., D.T. Stuss, A. Guzman, G. Lafleche, and J. Willmer. (1996). Diagnosis of dementia: methods for interpretation of scores of 5 neuropsychological tests. *Arch Neurol* 53:1043–1054.

Petersen, R.C. (2000). Aging, mild cognitive impairment, and Alzheimer's disease. *Dementia* 18:789–805.

Petersen, R.C., G.E. Smith, R.J. Ivnik, E.G. Tangalos, D.J. Schaid, S.N. Thibodeau, E. Kokmen, S.C. Waring, and L.T. Kurland. (1995). Apolipoprotein E status as a predictor of the development of Alzheimer's disease in memory-impaired individuals. *JAMA* 273:1274–1278.

Petersen R.C., G.E. Smith, S.C. Waring, R.J. Ivnik, E.G. Tangalos, and E. Kokmen. (1999). Mild cognitive impairment. *Arch Neurol* 56:303–308.

Reifler, B.V. (1997). Pre-dementia. *JAGS* 45:776–777.

Reischies, F.M., and R. Hellweg. (2000). Prediction of deterioration in mild cognitive disorder in older age: neuropsychological and neurochemical parameters of dementia diseases. *Comprehensive Psychiatry* 41:66–75.

Salthouse, T.A. (1996). The processing-speed theory of adult age differences in cognition. *Psychol Rev* 103:403–428.

Sliwinski, M., and H. Buschke. (1997). Processing speed and memory in aging and dementia. *J Gerontol Psychol Sci* 52B:308–318.

Sliwinski, M., H. Buschke, W.F. Stewart, D. Masur, and R.B. Lipton. (1997). The effect of dementia risk factors on comparative and diagnostic selective reminding norms. *J Int Neuropsychol Soc* 3:317–326.

Smith G.E., R.C. Petersen, J.E. Parisi, R.J. Ivnik, E. Kokmen, E.G. Tangalos, and S. Waring. (1996). Definition, course, and outcome of mild cognitive impairment. *Aging Neuropsychol Cognition* 3:141–147.

Sui, A.L. (1991). Screening for dementia and investigating its causes. *Ann Internal Med* 115:122–132.

CHAPTER 6

Magnetic Resonance Imaging

CLIFFORD R. JACK JR.

A number of different modalities are used for clinical imaging, and these can be grouped on the basis of the specific property of brain tissue measured as follows:

1. Gross anatomy and structure: MRI and CT
2. Biochemistry: MR spectroscopy
3. Glucose or oxygen metabolism: PET
4. Receptor density: PET
5. Cerebral blood flow: SPECT, MRI, PET
6. Tissue microstructure characterization: MRI–Magnetization Transfer, MRI–Diffusion-Weighted Imaging, MRI–Relaxometry
7. Functional task activation: MRI, PET

This chapter will be limited to a discussion of MR-based techniques used in the study of aging and dementia, specifically: anatomic MRI; ^{1}HMR spectroscopy; diffusion-weighted imaging (DWI); measures of regional cerebral blood flow and volume; and functional activation. The areas of emphasis in this chapter reflect the fact that the majority of the published literature in this area has focused on anatomic MRI.

The theme of this book is the interface between normal aging and dementia—specifically Alzheimer's disease. To relate the current imaging literature to this theme, it is helpful to consider that the motivation for imaging patients with dementia or patients at risk for dementia can be considered under three conceptual headings: diagnosis and characterization, staging, and monitoring disease progression. This chapter focuses on MR studies of diagnosis and characterization. Traditionally, imaging has been employed as a diagnostic tool in demented patients to exclude potentially treatable structural causes of dementia such as hydrocephalus, tumor, or subdural hematoma. Imaging has also traditionally been used to aid in the differential diagnosis of dementia; for example, identification of multiple areas of cerebral infarction would suggest a vascular contribution to the dementia. Investigators have also sought to identify positive imaging criteria for AD. More recently, the use of imaging has been extended to the early diagnosis of AD and identification of at-risk patients who are likely to convert to AD in the future.

DIAGNOSIS AND CHARACTERIZATION

Anatomic MRI

Relationship between MRI and Pathology of Alzheimer's Disease

Major pathologic features that characterize AD include senile plaques, neurofibrillary tangles, decreased synaptic density, neuron loss, and atrophy relative to age-matched controls (Tomlinson et al., 1970; Terry et al., 1981, 1991; Hyman et al., 1984; Price et al., 1991; Braak and Braak, 1994). The presumed pathologic basis of this atrophy is loss of neurons and decreased synaptic density. Cerebral atrophy identifiable with MRI seems to most closely parallel the distribution of neuronal pathology (versus the distribution of senile plaques). It is well established that the neurofibrillary pathology of AD begins in the transentorhinal area and then progresses in a stereotypical hierarchical fashion next to the hippocampus, to adjacent medial temporal lobe limbic areas, to neocortical association areas, and lastly to primary sensory and motor areas (Braak and Braak, 1991; Braak et al., 1993).

Assessment and Measurement of Cerebral Atrophy by MRI: Methodologic Considerations

Different approaches have been employed to assess brain size with anatomic MRI. Measures of atrophy can be divided into those that assess global or hemispheric atrophy and those that assess regional atrophy—that is, atrophy in specific portions of the brain. Methods for assessing atrophy can be divided into two general categories: visual ranking of scans, and formal quantitative measures of particular anatomic features. Visual ranking of cerebral atrophy represents an extension of the clinical practice of neuroradiology in which the severity of cerebral atrophy is commonly graded as mild, moderate, or severe. In its most rigorous implementation, visual ranking of scans for research purposes is accomplished by collecting a battery of example cases that represent the categories of atrophy into which the study scans will be grouped (Davis et al., 1992; Bryan et al., 1994). For example, each study scan may be assigned to one of four levels of atrophy—none, mild, moderate, or severe. For this type of visual ranking approach, a panel of expert readers is generally employed to rank the individual study scans, and quality control is assessed by monitoring measures of inter- and intrarater consistency in ranking scans.

The second general approach to evaluating cerebral atrophy is quantitative. Quantitative measures can be characterized as linear, area, or volumetric (DeCarli et al., 1990). Examples of linear measurements are the width of the frontal horns, third ventricle, various cortical sulci, and medial temporal lobe, as well as the interuncal distance. Examples of area measurements are measurements of the area of the lateral ventricles, frontal horn, third ventricle, corpus callosum, and hippocampus. Because the brain and cerebrospinal function (CSF) spaces are morphologically complicated three-dimensional structures, one might assume that greater accuracy would be found with a volume measurement than with a simpler linear or area measurement.

Cerebral atrophy is a negative phenomenon that does not lend itself to traditional positive counting methods (for example, counting the number of the senile plaques or neurofibrillary tangles). Therefore, cerebral atrophy must be characterized as a loss of tissue (or enlargement of the CSF spaces) relative to an appropriate group of elderly control individuals (Jack et al., 1992).

A common objective of imaging research studies is to identify a quantitative imaging measure that will separate appropriate elderly controls from cases. The objective is to isolate the relationship between a quantitative brain measure and the presence or absence of disease. However, at least three other important variables affect brain volume measurements in any individual: age, gender, and head size (head size being a surrogate for height or body habitus). To evaluate brain volume measurements in individual, elderly subjects, these measurements must be adjusted for age, gender, and head size and then referenced to an appropriate control population (Jack et al., 1989). The approach we have used is a W score—a covariate adjusted Z score (Jack et al., 1997). The volumes in each patient are converted to normal deviates with respect to age, head size, and gender-specific percentiles in elderly controls.

Overview of Types of Clinical Studies

Different types of clinical studies have been performed in an attempt to validate the usefulness of MRI-based imaging measurements for the diagnosis of AD. The published literature on this subject can be divided into five categories, depending on the study design employed. These categories are (1) cross-sectional case-control comparisons in which the cases are patients with clinically established AD; (2) cross-sectional case-control comparisons in which the cases are patients with very mild or early AD; (3) cross-sectional case-control comparisons in which the "cases" represent individuals who are at elevated risk for developing AD, but who at the time of the study do not meet established criteria for the diagnosis of AD; (4) longitudinal cohort studies in which an imaging study is performed at baseline in a cohort of individuals who are at higher risk for developing AD. The ability of an imaging measurement to predict which members of the cohort will and which will not develop AD is assessed; and (5) longitudinal cohort studies in which measures of the rates of change in MRI are assessed as potential biomarkers of disease progression.

The five types of clinical studies are listed here in ascending hierarchical rank order in terms of their significance in validating an imaging test as an early diagnostic marker of AD. Cross-sectional case-control comparisons in patients with clinically well-established AD constitute the least convincing evidence of the ability of an imaging test to make an early diagnosis of AD, whereas longitudinal prediction of the risk of developing AD in pre-morbid at-risk patients constitutes the most convincing demonstration of the utility of an imaging test for early diagnosis. The complexity of study design increases as one ascends the hierarchical rank order. And, not surprisingly, the number of published studies decreases as one ascends hierarchical rank order.

Cross-Sectional Case-Control Structural MRI Studies of Clinically Established Alzheimer's Disease

The initial step in identifying imaging markers that might be useful for the early diagnosis of AD is to establish that a significant difference in an imaging measure exists between patients with clinically established AD and age-matched elderly controls. An imaging test that is significantly different between controls and patients with established AD may not necessarily be useful at all for the early diagnosis of AD. However, imaging markers that are not different between controls and established AD patients are very unlikely to be useful for early diagnosis. Much of the published literature to date on the use of imaging for the diagnosis of AD has been based on this study design (Rusinek et al., 1991; Murphy et al., 1993; DeCarli et al., 1994, 1995; Lyoo et al., 1997; Tanabe et al., 1997; Bracco et al., 1999; Sencakova et al., 2001). While a number of different radiographic features have been assessed, recent interest has focused on the hippocampus or other medial temporal lobe structures with the intention of identifying markers of early disease. The rationale for the focus on the medial temporal lobe has been (*1*) medial temporal lobe limbic structures, particularly the hippocampus, play a central role in memory function; (*2*) memory impairment is the clinical hallmark of AD; and (*3*) modern MRI can precisely depict medial temporal lobe neuroanatomy. Approaches include visual ranking of the size of the hippocampus or peri-hippocampal CSF spaces, linear measurements of the inter-uncal distance, linear measurements of the medium thickness of the medial temporal lobe, area measurements of the hippocampus, and volume measurements of the hippocampus or other named medial temporal lobe limbic structures (Seab et al., 1988; Kesslak et al., 1991; Jack et al., 1992; Pearlson et al., 1992; Scheltens et al., 1992; Early et al., 1993; Howieson et al., 1993; Killiany et al., 1993; Lehtovirta et al., 1995; Maunoury et al., 1996; de Leon et al., 1997; Juottonen et al., 1999). The optimal approach is controversial, and generally each group advocates their own approach. The sensitivity and specificity with which controls can be separated from patients with established clinical AD has varied among different published studies. The ability of an imaging measurement to separate controls from AD patients clearly depends on the inclusion criteria used for selecting both the control subjects and the AD patients. In any particular study, the younger and healthier the control subjects and the more severely impaired the AD group, the better the diagnostic separation between controls and the AD patients.

Cross-Sectional Case-Control Structural MRI Studies of Early Alzheimer's Disease

The clinical studies described in this section consist of a comparison of controls to patients with clinically diagnosed AD whose mean Mini-Mental State Examination (MMSE) score was ≥ 22. Although this represents an arbitrary cutoff, the MMSE score is almost universally used and therefore defining "early" AD by MMSE ≥ 22 is at least operationally feasible. In most published anatomic MRI studies of early AD, some assessment of medial temporal lobe atrophy has been employed as the imaging metric. This includes visual ranking (mild, moderate, severe) of medial temporal lobe atrophy (de Leon et al., 1996), formal measures of hippocampal volume (Convit et al., 1993; Lehericy et al., 1994; Laakso et al., 1995, 1998), combinations of medial temporal and extratemporal measures (Murphy et al., 1993; Frisoni et al., 1996), and combinations of different named medial temporal lobe structures (Killiany et al., 1993).

In our own study of anatomic MRI measurements in early AD, we performed MRI-based volumetric measurements of the hippocampus, parahippocampal gyrus, and amygdala in 126 cognitively normal elderly control subjects and 94 patients with probable AD (Jack et al., 1997). The diagnosis of AD was made according to NINCDS-ADRDA criteria, and disease severity was categorized by clinical dementia (CDR) scores. Patients with CDR 0.5 were classified as very mild, and the mean MMSE score of this group was 22. We also included a group of AD patients with CDR score of 1, and a third AD patient group with CDR score of 2. The volume of each medial temporal lobe structure was significantly smaller in AD patients than in control subjects ($p < .001$). Of the different medial temporal lobe measures, the total hippocampal volume was best at discriminating control subjects from AD patients. The mean hippocampal volumes for AD patients relative to control subjects by severity of disease were as follows: CDR 0.5 AD, -1.75 SD below the control mean; CDR 1 AD, -1.99 SD below the control mean; and CDR 2 AD, -2.22 SD below the control mean. We therefore observed an increase in the difference between controls and AD patients as the severity of the impairment increased. The most significant finding, however, was the ability of hippocampal volume measurements to discriminate between control subjects and AD patients with very mild disease. Some 97.2% of all CDR 0.5 AD patients had hippocampal volumes below the fiftieth percentile of normal. These data demonstrated that MRI volume measurements of hippocampal atrophy are a sensitive marker of the pathology of AD early in the disease.

Cross-Sectional Case-Control Structural MRI Studies of Prodromal or At-Risk Patients

Several groups have performed cross-sectional studies comparing anatomic MRI measurements in controls to subjects at risk or in the prodromal phase of AD. "At risk" is defined as individuals who at the time of the study do not meet clinical criteria for AD but are at increased risk for developing AD in the future. For example, individuals who carry the $\varepsilon4$ allele of apolipoprotein E. Patients with a mild cognitive impairment (MCI), or patients with an age-associated memory impairment (AAMI), are considered by many to be in the prodromal phase of the disease.

For the most part, published studies find the degree of atrophy in MCI patients lies between normals and AD (De Santi et al., 2001; Dickerson et al., 2001; Du et al., 2001). Convit et al., (1995) measured a number of temporal lobe areas in a group of 27 normal elderly subjects, and 22 individuals who they termed "minimally impaired." It is not clear whether the group they described as "minimally impaired" met formal criteria for either MCI or AAMI; nonetheless, they were described as being at risk for future development of AD on the basis of neuropsychological criteria. Convit et al. (1995) found that the hippocampus was the only temporal lobe structure that differed significantly between the control and the minimally impaired group. Parnetti et al. (1996) studied six AD, six AAMI, and six cognitively normal elderly subjects and found lower hippocampal volume in the AAMI and probable AD groups than in the controls. Conversely, Soinennen et al. (1994) measured hippocampal and amygdala volume in 16 AAMI subjects and 16 controls and did not find a significant volume difference between the patient and control groups.

We tested the hypothesis that MRI-based measurements of the entorhinal cortex are more sensitive than are measurements of hippocampal volume in discriminating among three clinical groups: controls, patients with MCI, and patients with clinically diagnosed probable AD (Xu et al., 2000). The motivation for this study was the following. Although MRI-based measurements of hippocampal atrophy have been shown to be a sensitive indicator of the early pathologic degeneration of the medial temporal lobe in AD, AD pathology first appears in the transentorhinal cortex, not in the hippocampus. Therefore, entorhinal measurements theoretically should be more sensitive to the very earliest structural manifestations of AD that might be present in the prodromal phase who were destined to convert to AD. We studied 30 controls, 30 MCI patients, and 30 AD patients who were matched between clinical groups on age, gender, and education (Xu et al., 2000). All underwent a standardized MRI-imaging protocol, from which we made measurements of hippocampal volume, entorhinal cortex, and the cumulative length of the medial border of the entorhinal cortex. Pairwise intergroup differences ($p <$ .01) were found for all MRI measurements and between all groups, with the exception of the cumulative length of the entorhinal cortex, which did not differentiate controls from MCI patients. Greater atrophy was present in ADs than in MCIs, and more in MCIs than ADs than in normal controls. This atrophy ranking matches the relative cognitive performance of the three groups, control > MCI > AD (Fig. 6–1, 6–2, 6–3). While the hippocampal and entorhinal cortex volume measurements provide slightly better intergroup discrimination than the entorhinal distance measurement, overall differences in discriminating ability among the three MRI measurements were minor. We con-

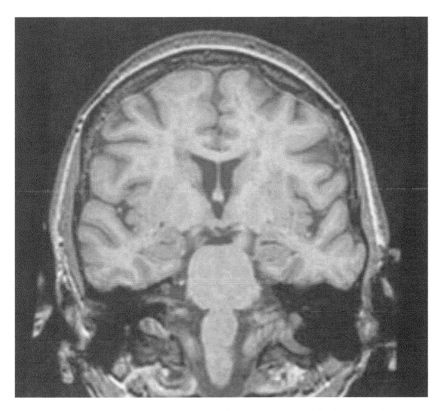

Figure 6–1. *Normal control.* Coronal MRI in a cognitively normal 70-year-old woman. Note the relative absence of cerebral atrophy relative to the patients in Figures 6–2 and 6–3.

clude that, despite the theoretical rationale for the superiority of entorhinal measurements in early AD and prodromal patients (i.e., MCIs), we found MRI measurements of the hippocampus and entorhinal cortex were approximately equivalent in intergroup discrimination. Measurements of the hippocampus may be preferable because the MRI depiction of the boundaries of the entorhinal cortex can be obscured by anatomic ambiguity, image artifact, or both.

Longitudinal Structural MRI Studies Using Imaging to Predict Development of Alzheimer's Disease

The next category of clinical studies to consider are those that actually document the ability of an imaging measurement to predict the future development of AD. By definition, these studies

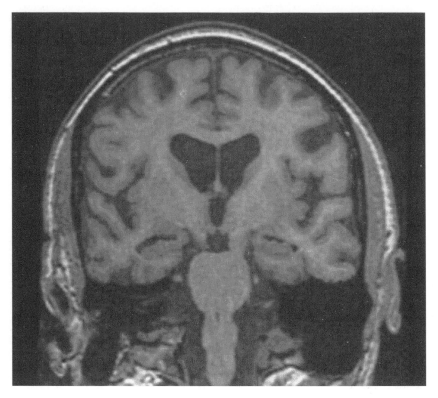

Figure 6–2. *Mild cognitive impairment (MCI)*. Coronal MRI in 77-year-old man with MCI. The degree of atrophy (particularly in the medial temporal regions bilaterally) is of intermediate severity between the normal control in Figure 6–1 and the AD patient in Figure 6–3.

are longitudinal in nature. A group of patients who have a higher risk for developing AD (for example, on the basis of extreme old age, having MCI, or having a particular genotype) but who at the time of enrollment do not meet criteria for AD are followed longitudinally.

Several published studies fall under the category of using a single baseline anatomic MRI measurement at the time of enrollment to predict subsequent conversion to AD. Our own work in this area employed MRI-based hippocampal volume in patients with MCI to predict future conversion to AD (Jack et al., 1999). Eighty consecutive patients who met criteria for the diagnosis of MCI were recruited from the Mayo Clinic Alzheimer's

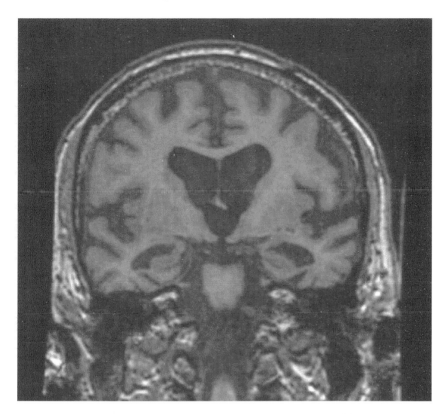

Figure 6–3. *Alzheimer's disease (AD)*. Coronal MRI in 77-year-old man with AD. The degree of atrophy (particularly in the medial temporal regions bilaterally) is of greater severity than the MCI patient in Figure 6–2 and substantially greater severity than the normal control in Figure 6–1.

Disease Center/Alzheimer's Disease Patient Registry (Table 6–1). At entry into the study, each patient received an MRI examination of the head, from which the volumes of both hippocampi were measured. Patients were followed longitudinally with approximately annual clinical and cognitive assessments. The primary endpoint was the crossover of individual MCI patients to the clinical diagnosis of AD during longitudinal clinical follow-up. During the period of longitudinal observation, which averaged 32.6 months, 27 of the 80 MCI patients became demented. Hippocampal atrophy at baseline was significantly associated with crossover from MCI to AD (relative risk 0.69, p = .015) (Fig. 6–4).

Table 6–1. Characterization of Patients with Mild Cognitive Impairment

	N	Age[a] (mean ± SD)	Male	MMSE[b] (mean ± SD)	DRS[c] (mean ± SD)	Education (mean ± SD)	APOEε4[d]	Follow-up in months[e] (mean ± SD)	Crossover to AD
Hippocampal W Score ≥ 0	13	79.6 ± 6.1	6 (46.2%)	26.2 ± 2.3	127.3 ± 6.9	11.7 ± 3.1	4 (30.8%)	42.4 ± 15.4	2 (15%)
Hippocampal W Score < 0	54	78.3 ± 6.4	23 (42.6%)	26.7 ± 2.3	127.6 ± 9.4	13.3 ± 3.5	19 (35.2%)	32.5 ± 18.4	19 (35%)
Hippocampal W Score ≤ −2.5	13	73.7 ± 8.2	4 (30.8%)	25.3 ± 3.4	126.5 ± 8.6	13.7 ± 3.1	6 (46.2%)	23.3 ± 10.7	6 (46%)
Total	80	77.7 ± 6.8	33 (41.25%)	26.4 ± 2.5	127.4 ± 8.8	13.1 ± 3.4	9 (36.25%)	32.6 ± 17.6	27 (34%)

Source: Adapted from Jack et al. (1999).

[a]Age at time of MRI study, i.e., at time patient entered into the study.

[b]Mini-Mental State Examination score when patient entered the study. Maximum score is 30.

[c]Dementia Rating Scale score when patient entered the study. Maximum score is 144.

[d]Numbers in this column represent the number of patients in each group who were carriers of *APOE* genotypes that are known to confer an increased risk of AD, ε3/4 and 4/4. Patients (*n* = 6) with ε2/4 were not included.

[e]Follow-up is from time of entry into study to conversion to AD in those patients who crossed over.

Note: A hippocampal W score ≥ 0, is ≥ the expected mean for controls. A W score ≤ −2.5, is < the first percentile for controls.

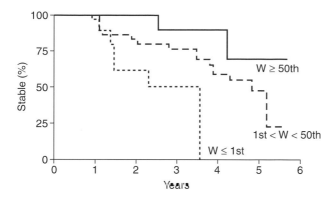

Figure 6–4. *Hippocampal volumes predicting conversion from MCI to AD.* Kaplan-Meyer curves of three groups of MCI subjects: (*1*) those whose hippocampal W scores at baseline were greater or equal to the expected mean (i.e., the 50th percentile) for normal controls (n = 13); (*2*) those whose hippocampal W scores were between the control mean and the 1st percentile of controls (n = 54); (*3*) those whose hippocampal W scores were less than the 1st percentile of normal controls (n – 13).

When hippocampal volume was entered into bivariate models—using age, postmenopausal estrogen replacement, standard neuropsychological tests, apolipoprotein E, genotype, history of ischemic heart disease, and hypertension—the relative risks were not substantially different from that found univariately, and the associations between hippocampal volume and crossover remained significant. We conclude that in older patients with MCI, hippocampal atrophy determined by premorbid MRI-based volume measurements is predictive of subsequent crossover to AD.

Vissur et al. (1999), Laasko (2000), and Killiany (2000) have published studies documenting the association between baseline medial temporal volume measurements and subsequent conversion to AD in at risk individuals. Earlier, de Leon et al. (1993) employed visual rating of hippocampal atrophy at baseline to predict subsequent crossover.

Serial Structural MRI Studies as Biomarkers of Disease Progression

We have assessed the correlation between the rate of hippocampal atrophy and the change in cognitive status of controls, MCIs, and AD patients over time (Jack et al., 2000). We identified 129 subjects from the Mayo Clinic AD Research Center/AD Patient Registry who met established criteria for normal controls, MCI, or probable AD both at entry and at the time of a subsequent clinical follow-up evaluation about 3 years later. Each subject underwent an MRI examination of the head at the time of the initial assessment and at the time of the follow-up clinical assessment. The annualized percentage change in hippocampal volume was computed. Controls and MCI patients either could remain cognitively stable or could decline to a lower functioning group over the period of observation. This study allowed us to test the hypothesis that the annualized rates of hippocampal atrophy differ as a function of both baseline and change in clinical group membership (control, MCI, or AD). This also is equivalent to testing the hypothesis that the rates of hippocampal atrophy were valid biomarkers of disease progression. The mean annualized rates of hippocampal atrophy by follow-up clinical group were control-stable, 1.73%, control-decliner, 2.81%; MCI-stable, 2.55%; MCI-decliner, 3.69%; and AD, 3.5%. Within the control and MCI groups, those who declined to a lower functioning clinical group over the course of follow-up had a significantly greater rate of volume loss than those who remained clinically stable.

Kaye et al. (1997) measured serial hippocampal and parahippocampal volumes in 30 individuals who at baseline were cognitively normal but were at risk for developing AD on the basis of extreme old age. A total of 12 of the 30 experienced significant cognitive decline over the period of observation. These data were obtained from a longitudinal study of the "oldest old," and the mean age of the 12 decliners was 90 years, with several individuals having an age in excess of 100 years. Kaye et al. (1997) found more rapid volume loss in the parahippocampal gyrus (but not the hippocampus) in decliners than in the stable elderly individuals.

Fox and colleagues (Fox et al., 1996; Fox and Freeborough, 1997) have pioneered the measurement of change in global cerebral volume from serial MRI studies (Fox et al., 2000, 2001). They studied a group of individuals who at baseline were asymptomatic, but who were at risk for future development of AD due to a family history of autosomal dominant early-onset (less than 65 years) Alzheimer's disease (Fox et al., 1999b). They studied

28 at-risk individuals and 26 age-matched cognitively normal volunteers in this manner. Five at-risk patients developed symptoms of cognitive decline during follow-up and subsequently progressed to fulfill established criteria for probable AD. The median rate of atrophy was 1.5% per year in these five individuals, which was significantly greater ($p < .0005$) than the median rate of 0.2% in the control group and also significantly greater than the median rate of 0.1% per year in the 23 at-risk individuals who remained asymptomatic. While minor overlap in the annualized rates of whole brain atrophy was present between the members of the decliner group and the at-risk unaffected group, there was no overlap between the decliner group and the normal controls.

MR Spectroscopy

The primary ^{1}HMRS abnormalities that have been associated with AD are a decrease in N-acetyl aspartate (NAA) and an elevation in myoinositol (MI) (Klunk et al., 1992; Miller et al., 1993; Shonk 1995b). NAA is found in neurons, and a decrease in NAA follows logically from the neuron loss associated with AD. NAA has also been proposed as a marker of neuron viability, as declines in NAA are reversible in some situations—for example, reversible ischemia or epilepsy (Hugg et al., 1996). This has led some investigators to advocate that a decline in NAA may precede cell loss in AD, and thus ^{1}HMRS may be a more sensitive marker of early disease than is anatomic MRI. Myoinositol is located primarily in astrocytes. It is higher in AD and Down syndrome, but the reason for this elevation is not entirely clear. One intriguing possibility is that the observed elevation in myoinositol is a function of the glial activation associated with neuritic plaques (Shonk and Ross, 1995b; Kantarci, 2000).

While the number of ^{1}HMRS publications is far smaller than the number of anatomic MRI studies, a convincing body of literature exists, documenting significant differences in certain ^{1}HMRS metabolites between controls and patients with established AD. As is the case with anatomic MR studies, for the most part the published ^{1}HMRS literature has employed a cross-sectional case versus control comparison design. In the published literature, the metabolites that consistently differ between case and control sample groups are NAA and MI (Klunk et al., 1992;

Miller et al., 1993; Meyerhoff et al., 1994; Shonk and Ross, 1995; Tedeschi et al., 1996; Schuff et al., 1997, 1998; Catani et al., 2001; Huang et al., 2001). Elevations in lactate and choline have also been described in AD, but these results have not been found consistently.

Fewer spectroscopic studies have been performed comparing control subjects to at-risk subjects. We compared ^{1}HMRS findings in the superior temporal lobe, posterior cingulate gyri, and medial occipital lobe among 21 patients with MCI, 21 patients with probable AD, and 63 elderly controls (Kantarci et al., 2000b). These areas are known to be involved at different neurofibrillary pathologic stages of AD. The NAA/creatine ratios were significantly lower in AD patients than in both MCI and normal control subjects in the left superior temporal and posterior cingulate volumes of interest. MI/Cr ratios measured from the posterior cingulate volume of interest (VOI) were significantly higher in both MCI and AD patients than in controls. These findings suggest that the initial ^{1}HRMS change in the pathologic progression of AD is an increase in MI/Cr. A decrease in NAA/Cr develops later in the disease.

Pareneti et al. (1996) acquired ^{1}HMRS spectra in six patients with AD, six AAMI subjects, and six controls. They found significantly greater MI in AD patients than in controls and significantly lower NAA in AD patients and AAMI subjects than in controls.

Diffusion-Weighted Imaging

Diffusion-weighted MRI (DWI) is an imaging technique that is sensitive to the microscopic diffusion of water molecules in biologic tissue (Stejskal and Tanner, 1965; LeBihan et al., 1986). Cell membranes and intracellular structures act to impede the diffusion of water molecules, whereas disruption of cell membranes or normal intracellular structure increases the diffusivity of water. Cell death and reactive astrocytosis expand the size of the extracellular compartment and thus increase water diffusion. Because the direction of water diffusion can be measured relative to the orthogonal geometric axes of the MR magnet, the degree of geometric isotropy of water diffusion can also be measured.

Several cross-sectional case-control studies have been published; they assess the ability of DWI to differentiate between controls and clinically established AD patients (Hanyu et al., 1997, 1998; Sandson et al., 1999). While published results are not entirely consistent, in general, an increase in diffusion values has been seen in selected regions of interest in AD patients compared to controls. Results on diffusion asymmetry are less consistent, with some studies reporting increased diffusion asymmetry in AD, while in other studies diffusion asymmetry has not been a prominent feature of AD.

We recently compared the apparent diffusion coefficient (ADC) and the anisotropy indices (AI) obtained from frontal, parietal, temporal, occipital, anterior, and posterior cingulate white matter, thalamic and hippocampal regions of interest in 21 probable AD, 19 MCI patients, and 55 normal aging elderly controls without evidence of cognitive impairment (Kantarci et al., 2000a, 2001). The major finding of this study was higher levels of hippocampal ADC in both MCI and AD patients than in controls. Most important, hippocampal ADC was significantly different between controls and MCI patients, indicating that a higher level of hippocampal ADC may reflect early ultrastructural changes in the progression of Alzheimer's pathology.

Sandson et al. (1999) found an elevation in the ADC of the parietal white matter in patients with established AD over that in controls. Our findings agree with this observation. Hanyu et al. (1998) found an elevation in ADC in the temporal stem in patients with established AD over that in controls, and our data agree with this finding as well.

MR Perfusion

A characteristic bilateral temporal-parietal decrease in cerebral blood flow has been well documented using nuclear medicine techniques in AD (Jagust et al., 1987; Johnson et al., 1987). Gonzales et al. (1995) studied clinically established AD patients with dynamic bolus tracking MRI. The technique provides images of dynamic-contrast susceptibility weighting that mirror region blood volume distribution. These dynamic-contrast susceptibility images were compared to [18]FDG PET studies in the same patients, and a high degree of concordance was found. Gonzales et al. (1995) concluded that the characteristic bilateral temporal parietal perfusion/metabolism defects seen with PET/SPECT in AD can be identified with dynamic contrast susceptibility MRI techniques. Harris et al. (1998) used a similar MR technique and compared the results to SPECT measures of cerebral perfusion. The dynamic susceptibility contrast MR approach compared favorably to SPECT in distinguishing controls from patients with established AD. More recently, Alsop et al. (2000) employed an MR measurement of cerebral perfusion using an arterial-spin-labeling technique. They found significant perfusion differences between controls and patients with established AD in the temporal, parietal, frontal, and posterior cingulate cortices. The advantage of this approach is that no contrast injection is required, and thus the technique is completely noninvasive.

Functional Activation

Medial temporal lobe functional activation in response to declarative memory paradigms have been demonstrated in normal young volunteers by several investigators using functional MRI (Stern et al., 1996; Gabrieli et al., 1997; Rombouts et al., 1997, 1999; Fernandez et al., 1998; Dolan and Fletcher, 1999; Strange et al., 1999). The pathology of AD results in specific neurocognitive deficits. The initial, and most pronounced, cognitive deficit typically is of declarative memory. A functional MRI examination of declarative memory should serve as a functional medial temporal lobe "stress test." This approach has significant theoretical appeal because functional changes in response to early AD pathology should precede the gross anatomic changes measured by structural MRI (Corkin, 1998). Functional MRI activation studies in aging and dementia have been performed in small numbers of AD patients at a few research sites (Small et al., 1999; Smith et al., 1999b). Investigators have been able to demonstrate decreased functional activation in the medial temporal region in patients with AD when compared to age-matched controls. This is an area of research that is just beginning to unfold, and it is being pursued at a number of research sites. Significant technical problems remain to be solved, however, including functional MRI artifacts due to head motion, artifacts due to magnetic susceptibility effects in the medial-basal temporal lobe, potential decreased vascular responsiveness in elderly persons, and design of appropriate paradigms for medial temporal functional MRI activation that can be reliably performed by elderly and impaired subjects.

CAVEATS FOR IMAGING DIAGNOSIS AND CHARACTERIZATION OF ALZHEIMER'S DISEASE

Successful versus Pathologic Aging

Cerebral atrophy and leukoaraiosis (i.e., white-matter microangiopathy) increase in both prevalence and severity with advancing age and therefore can justifiably be considered a feature of normal aging. But atrophy both radiographically and pathologically is the hallmark of Alzheimer's disease and therefore cannot justifiably be labeled "normal." This has led to a distinction between successful (or healthy) aging versus pathologic aging. From an imaging perspective, aging can conceptually be divided into three categories: (1) healthy or successful aging, which implies the absence of cerebral pathology; (2) usual aging, which is the presence of cerebral pathology to a degree that is commonly found in members of the general population for a given age bracket; and (3) pathologic aging, which may be defined as cerebral pathology that is more severe than commonly found in members of the general population within a given age bracket.

The preceding discussion raises two issues that are relevant when developing imaging criteria to distinguish among healthy aging, usual aging, and pathologic aging. First, cerebral atrophy exists in a continuous distribution across the general population. In practice, forcing the continuous distribution of brain volumes found in the general population into these three theoretical categories is done by establishing threshold or cutoff points in a continuous distribution. The division of a population on the basis of cerebral atrophy into the categories of healthy aging, usual aging, and pathologic aging is therefore somewhat arbitrary. Second, the definitions of usual aging and pathologic aging change with advancing age. Because cerebral atrophy becomes more prevalent and more severe with advancing age, a level of cerebral atrophy that might be labeled pathologic in a 60-year-old may well fall into the range for usual aging in a 90-year-old.

The control groups employed in the vast majority of imaging studies in aging and dementia have recruited individuals who could best be classified as usual aging. The control subjects include individuals with some degree of cerebral pathology (atrophy, leukoaraiosis, etc.), and it is likely that most control populations include some individuals with preclinical or presymptomatic AD, who at some point in the future will declare themselves clinically. On the one hand, this is appropriate because a clinically useful imaging measurement should be able to separate a typical cognitively intact elderly person from a patient with clinically evident AD. On the other hand, by labeling some degree of cerebral atrophy "normal," the efficacy of any imaging measure of cerebral atrophy in discriminating controls from AD patients is diminished. The problem of contamination of control samples with individuals who have presymptomatic AD is common to many case-control studies in this field, not just MRI studies, and it is difficult to address.

Specificity

A significant limitation of imaging in the diagnosis of neurodegenerative disorders is the lack of specificity for the molecular events that lead to cell death. This lack of molecular specificity is not restricted to MRI-based techniques. A similar lack of specificity would also be expected with nuclear medicine–based measurements of glucose or oxygen metabolism, or blood flow.

ADDITIONAL USES FOR IMAGING

To this point, this chapter has been devoted largely to a discussion of the use of imaging for the diagnosis and characterization of AD, specifically early and preclinical AD. The potential clinical use of imaging should be mentioned, however, in two other contexts: staging of disease severity and as a biomarker of disease progression. A number of anatomic imaging studies, including our own, have documented a close correlation between the severity of cerebral atrophy as measured with in vivo MRI and the severity of the cognitive deficit in AD patients (Deweer et al., 1995; Pantel et al., 1997; Petersen et al., 1998, 2000; Fox, 1999b; Smith et al., 1999a). The severity of the cognitive deficit in patients typically has been assessed with formal cognitive testing instruments.

More recently Bobinski et al. (2000) have undertaken a formal correlation between measurements of hippocampal volume from MRI exams done on postmortem brains and histologic measures of AD pathology. They found a highly significant correlation between postmortem MRI-defined hippocampal volume and histologically defined hippocampal area. They also found a significant correlation between the MR measures of hippocampal atrophy and histologic measures of cell loss.

Our own work in this area has consisted of correlation between premortem MRI, and postmortem assessments of Braak staging (Braak and Braak, 1991). We found a significant inverse correlation between hippocampal volume and Braak stage. These data, combined with those of Bobinski, indicate that MRI-defined hippocampal volume measurements represent a valid in vivo surrogate for the pathologic staging of AD (Jack et al., 2002).

While mentioned earlier, added emphasis should be placed on the use of imaging as a biomarker of progression of the disease. This is an area that to date has been studied, but has tremendous potential utility. In this setting, imaging studies are typically performed serially, and longitudinal measurements of the rate of change are made. This type of information is useful in two different contexts. First, the rate of change—for example, of brain volume—may be a useful adjunct for monitoring progression of the disease in individual patients either for purposes of clinical prognostication or to gauge the results from therapeutic intervention. Longitudinal measurements may also be useful as a means of comparing rates of change among different groups of subjects. The use of serial imaging measurements as a surrogate marker of drug efficacy in therapeutic trials is feasible (Jack et al., 1998; Fox et al., 2000).

Acknowledgments

Grateful appreciation to Brenda Maxwell for typing this manuscript. Supported by NIH-NIA-AG11378; AG16574; AG-08031; AG-06786; The DANA Foundation; The Alzheimer's Association.

References

Alsop, D.C., J.A. Detre, and M. Grossman. (2000). Assessment of cerebral blood flow in Alzheimer's disease by spin-labeled magnetic resonance imaging. *Ann Neurol* 47:93–100.

Bobinski, M., M.J. deLeon, J. Wegiel, and S. Desanti. (2000). The histological validation of post mortem magnetic resonance imaging-determined hippocampal volume in Alzheimer's disease. *Neuroscience* 95: 721–725.

Braak, H., and E. Braak. (1991). Neuropathological staging of Alzheimer-related changes. *Acta Neuropathol* 82:239–259.

Braak, H., and E. Braak. (1994). Morphological criteria for the recognition of Alzheimer's disease and the distribution pattern of cortical changes related to this disorder. *Neurobiol Aging* 15:355–356.

Braak, H., E. Braak, and J. Bohl. (1993). Staging of Alzheimer-related cortical destruction. Eur Neurol 33:403–408.

Bracco, L., C. Piccini, G. Manfredi, C. Fonda, and M. Falcini. (1999). Magnetic resonance measures in Alzheimer's disease: their utiligy in early diagnosis and evaluating disease progression. *Alzheimer Disease Associated Disorders* 13:157–164.

Bryan, R.N., T.A. Manolio, and L.D. Schertz. (1994). A method for using MR to evaluate the effects of cardiovascular disease on the brain: the Cardiovascular Health Study. *AJNR* 15:1625–1633.

Catani, M., A. Cherubini, and R. Howard. (2001). ^{1}H MR spectroscopy differentiates mild cognitive impairment from normal brain aging. *Neuroreport* 12(11):2315–2317.

Convit, A., M.J. de Leon, and J. Golomb. (1993). Hippocampal atrophy in early Alzheimer's disease: anatomic specificity and validation. *Psychiatric Q* 64:371–387.

Convit, A., M.H. de Leon, and C. Tarshish. (1995). Hippocampal volume losses in minimally impaired elderly. *Lancet* 345:266.

Corkin, S. (1998). Functional MRI for studying episodic memory in aging and Alzheimer's disease. *Geriatrics* 1:S13–15.

Davis, P.C., L. Gray, and M. Albert. (1992). The consortium to establish a registry for Alzheimer's disease (CERAD). Part III. Reliability of a standardized MRI evaluation of Alzheimer's disease. *Neurology* 42:1676–1680.

DeCarli, C., J.A. Kaye, B. Horwitz, and S.I. Rapoport. (1990). Critical analysis of the use of computer-assisted transverse axial tomography to study human brain in aging and dementia of the Alzheimer type. *Neurology* 40:872–883.

DeCarli, C., D.G.M. Murphy, and A.R. McIntosh. (1994). Discriminant analysis of Alzheimer's disease. *Arch Neurol* 51:1088–1089.

DeCarli, C., D.G.M. Murphy, and A.R. McIntosh. (1995). Discriminant analysis of MRI measures as a method to determine the presence of dementia of the Alzheimer type. *Psychiatry Res* 57(2):119–130.

de Leon, M.J., J. Golomb, and A.E. George. (1993). The radiologic prediction of Alzheimer disease: the atrophic hippocampal formation. *AJNR* 14:897–906.

de Leon, M.J., A. Convit, and A.E. George. (1996). In vivo structural studies of the hippocampus in normal aging and in incipient Alzheimer's disease. *Ann N Y Acad Sci* 777:1–13.

de Leon, M.J., A.E. George, and J. Golomb. (1997). Frequency of hippocampal formation atrophy in normal aging and Alzheimer's disease. *Neurobiol Aging* 18:1–11.

De Santi, S., M.J. de Leon, and H. Rusinek. (2001). Hippocampal formation glucose metabolism and volume losses in MCI and AD. *Neurobiol Aging* 22(4):529–539.

Deweer, B., S. Lehericy, and B. Pillon. (1995). Memory disorders in probable Alzheimer's disease: the role of hippocampal atrophy as shown with MRI. *Neurol Neurosurg Psychiatry* 58:590–597.

Dickerson, B.C., I. Goncharova, and M.P. Sullivan. (2001). MRI-derived entorhinal and hippocampal atrophy in incipient and very mild Alzheimer's disease. *Neurobiol Aging* 22(5):747–754.

Dolan, R.J., and P.F. Fletcher. (1999). Encoding and retrieval in human medial temporal lobes: an empirical investigation usign functional magnetic resonance imaging (fMRI). *Hippocampus* 9:25–34.

Du, A.T., N. Schuff, and D. Amend. (2001). Magnetic resonance imaging of the entorhinal cortex and hippocampus in mild cognitive impairment and Alzheimer's disease. *J Neurol Neurosurg Psychiatry* 71(4):431–432.

Early, B., P.R. Escalona, O.B. Boyko, and P.M. Doraiswamy. (1993). Interuncal distance measurements in healthy volunteers and in patients with Alzheimer Disease. *AJNR* 14:907–910.

Fernandez, G., H. Weyerts, and M. Schrader-Bolsche. (1998). Successful verbal encoding into episodic memory engages the posterior hippcampus: a parametrically analyzed functional magnetic resonance imaging study. *J Neurosci* 18:1841–1847.

Fox, N.C., and P.A. Freeborough. (1997). Brain atrophy progression measured from registered serial MRI: validation and application to Alzheimer's disease. *J Magnetic Resonance Imaging* 7:1069–1075.

Fox, N.C., P.A. Freeborough, and M.N. Rossor. (1996). Visualisation and quantification of rates of atrophy in Alzheimer's disease. *Lancet* 348: 94–97.

Fox, N.C., R.I. Scahill, W.R. Crum, and M.N. Rossor. (1999a). Correlation between rates of brain atrophy and cognitive decline in AD. *Neurology* 52:1687–1689.

Fox, N.C., E.K. Warrington, and M.N. Rossor. (1999b). Serial magnetic resonance imaging of cerebral atrophy in preclinial Alzheimer's disease. *Lancet* 353:2125.

Fox, N.C., S. Cousens, and R. Scahill. (2000). Using serial registered brain maganetic resonance imaging to measure disease progression in Alzheimer disease. *Arch Neurol* 57(3):339–443.

Fox, N.C., S. Cousens, and R. Scahill. (2000). Using serial registered brain magnetic resonance imaging to measure disease progression in Alzheimer disease: power calculations and estimates of sample size to detect treatment effects. *Arch Neurol* 57(3):339–344.

Fox, N.C., W.F. Crum, and R.I. Scahill. (2001). Imaging of onset and progression of Alzheimer's disease with voxel compression mapping of serial magnetic resonance images. *Lancet* 358:201–205.

Frisoni, G.B., A. Beltramello, and C. Weiss. (1996). Usefulness of simple measures of temporal lobe atrophy in probable Alzheimer's disease. *Dementia* 7:15–22.

Gabrieli, J.D., J.B. Brewer, J.E. Desmond, and G.H. Glover. (1997). Separate neural bases of two fundamental memory processes in the human medial temporal lobe. *Science* 276:264–266.

Gonzalez, R.G., A.J. Fischman, A.R. Guimaraes, and C.A. Carr. (1995). Functional MR in the evaluation of dementia: correlation of abnormal dynamic cerebral blood volume measurements with changes in cerebral metabolism on positron emission tomography with fludeoxyglucose F18. *AJNR* 16:1763–1770.

Hanyu, H., H. Shindo, D. Kakizaki, K. Abe, and T. Iwamoto. (1997). Increased water diffusion in cerebral white matter in Alzheimer's disease. *Gerontology* 43:343–351.

Hanyu, H., H. Sakurai, M. Takasaki, H. Shindo, and K. Abe. (1998). Diffusion weighted MR imaging of the hippocampus and temporal white matter in Alzheimer's disease. *J Neurol Sci* 156:195–200.

Harris, G.J., R.F. Lewis, A. Satlin, C.D. English, and T.M. Scott. (1998). Dynamic susceptibility contrast MR imaging of regional cerebral blood volume in Alzheimer disease: a promising alternative to nuclear medicine. *AJNR* 19:1727–1732.

Howieson, J., J.A. Kaye, L. Holm, and D. Howieson. (1993). Interuncal distance: marker of aging and Alzheimer disease. *AJNR* 14:647–650.

Huang, W., G.E. Alexander, and L. Chang. (2001). Brain metabolite concentration and dementia severity in Alzheimer's disease. A ^{1}H MRS study. *Neurology* 57:626–632.

Hugg, J.W., R.I. Kuziecky, and F.G. Gilliam. (1996). Normalization of contralateral metabolic function following temporal lobectomy demonstrated by ^{1}H magnetic resonance spectroscopic imaging. *Ann Neurol* 40:236–239.

Hyman, B.T., G.W. Van Hoesen, A.R. Damasio, and C.L. Barnes. (1984). Alzheimer's disease: cell-specific pathology isolates the hippocampal formation. *Science* 225:1168–1170.

Jack, C.R., Jr., C.K. Twomey, and A.R. Zinsmeister. (1989). Anterior temporal lobes and hippocampal formations: normative volumetric measurements for MR images in young adults. *Radiology* 172:549–554.

Jack, C.R., Jr., R.C. Petersen, and P.C. O'Brien. (1992). MR-based hippocampal volumetry in the diagnosis of Alzheimer's disease. *Neurology* 42:183–188.

Jack, C.R., Jr., R.C. Petersen, and Y.C. Xu. (1997). Medial temporal atrophy on MRI in normal aging and very mild Alzheimer's disease. *Neurology* 49:786–794.

Jack, C.R., Jr., R.C. Petersen, and Y. Xu. (1998). The rate of medial temporal lobe atrophy in typical aging and Alzheimer's disease. *Neurology* 51:993–999.

Jack, C.R., Jr., R.C. Petersen, and Y. Xu. (1999). Prediction of AD with MRI-based hippocampal volume in mild cognitive impairment. *Neurology* 52:1397–1403.

Jack, C.R., Jr., R.C. Petersen, Y. Xu, P.C. O'Brien, G.E. Smith, R.J. Ivnik, B.F. Boeve, E.G. Tangalos, and E. Kokmen. (2000). Rates of hippocampal atrophy in normal aging, mild cognitive impairment, and Alzheimer's disease. *Neurology* 55:484–489.

Jack, C.R., Jr., D.W. Dickson, J.E. Parisi, Y. Xu, R.H. Cha, P.C. O'Brien, S.D. Edland, G.E. Smith, B.F. Boeve, E.G. Tangalos, E. Kokmen, and R.C. Petersen. (2002). Antemortem MRI findings correlate with hippocampal neuropathology in typical aging and dementia. *Neurology* 58:750–757.

Jagust, W.J., T.F. Budinger, and B.R. Reed. (1987). The diagnosis of dementia with single photon emission computed tomography. *Arch Neurol* 44:258–262.

Johnson, K.A., S.T. Mueller, and T.M. Walshe. (1987). Cerebral perfusion imaging in Alzheimer's disease. *Arch Neurol* 44:165–168.

Juottonen, K., M. Laakso, K. Partanen, and H. Soinine. (1999). Comparative MR analysis of the entorhinal cortex and hippocampus in diagnosing Alzheimer Disease. *AJNR* 20:139–144.

Kantarci, J., C.R. Jack, Jr., Y.C. Xu, N.G. Campeau, P.C. O'Brien, G.E. Smith, R.J. Ivnik, B.F. Boeve, E. Kokmen, E.G. Tangalos, and R.C. Petersen. (2001). Mild cognitive impairment and Alzheimer's disease: regional diffusivity of water[1]. *Radiology* 219(1):101–107.

Kantarci, K., C.R. Jack, Jr., Y. Xu, N.G. Cmpeau, P.C. O'Brien, G.E. Smith, R.J. Ivnik, B.F. Boeve, E. Kokmen, E.G. Tangalos, and R.C. Petersen. (2000). Regional metabolic patterns in mild cognitive impairment and ad: A ^{1}H MRS study. *Neurology* 55(2):210–217.

Kaye, J.A., T. Swihart, D. Howieson, and A. Dame. (1997). Volume loss of the hippocampus and temporal lobe in healthy elderly persons destined to develop dementia. *Neurology* 48:1297–1304.

Kesslak, J.P., O. Nalcioglu, and C.W. Cotman. (1991). Quantification of magnetic resonance scans for hippocampal and parahippocampal atrophy in Alzheimer's disease. *Neurology* 41:51–54.

Killiany, R.J., M.B. Moss, and M.S. Albert. (1993). Temporal lobe regions on magnetic resonance imaging identify patients with early Alzheimer's disease. *Arch Neurol* 50:949–954.

Killany R.J., T. Gomez-Isla, and M. Moss. (2000). Use of structural Magnetic Resonance Imaging to predict who will get Alzheimer's disease. *Ann Neurol* 47:430–439.

Klunk, W.E., K. Panchalingam, and J. Moossy. (1992). *N*-acetyl-L-aspartate and other amino acid metabolites in Alzheimer's disease brain: a preliminary proton nuclear magnetic resonance study. *Neurology* 42:1578–1585.

Laakso, M.P., H. Soininen, and K. Partanen. (1995). Volumes of hippocampus, amygdala and frontal lobes in the MRI-based diagnosis of early Alzheimer's disease: correlation with memory functions. *J Neural Transmission* 9:73–86.

Laasko, M.P., H. Soinen, and K. Partanen. (1998). MRI of the hippocampus in Alzheimer's disease: sensitivity, specificity, and analysis of the incorrectly classified subjects. *Neurobiol Aging* 19(1), 23–3.

Laasko, M.P., M. Lehtovirta, and K. Partanen. (2000). Hippocampus in Alzheimer's disease: a 3-year follow-up MRI study. *Biol Psychiatry* 47(6): 557–561.

LeBihan, D., E. Breton, D. Lallemand, P. Grenier, and E. Cabanis. (1986). MR imaging of incoherent motions: application to diffusion and perfusion in neurologic disorders. *Radiology* 161:401–407.

Lehericy, S., M. Baulac, and J. Chiras. (1994). Amygdalohippocampal MR volume measurements in the early stages of Alzheimer disease. *AJNR* 15:927–937.

Lehtovirta, M., M.P. Laakso, and H. Soininen. (1995). Volumes of hippocampus, amygdala and frontal lobe in Alzheimer's patients with different apolipoprotein E genotypes. *Neuroscience* 67:65–72.

Lyoo, I.K., A. Satlin, C.K. Lee, and P.F. Renshaw. (1997). Regional atrophy of the corpus callosum in subjects with Alzheimer's disease and multi-infarct dementia. *Psychiatry Res* 74:63–72.

Maunoury, C., J.-L. Michot, and H. Caillet. (1996). Specificity of temporal amygdala atrophy in Alzheimer's disease: quantitative assessment with magnetic resonance imaging. *Dementia* 7:10–14.

Meyerhoff, D.J., S. MacKay, and J.-M. Constans. (1994). Axonal injury and membrain alterations in Alzheimer's disease suggested by in vivo proton magnetic resonance spectroscopic imaging. *Ann Neurol* 36:40–47.

Miller, B.L., R.A. Moats, and T. Shonk. (1993). Alzheimer disease: depiction of increased cerebral myo-inositol with proton MR spectroscopy. *Radiology* 187:433–437.

Murphy, D.G.M., C.D. DeCarli, and E. Daly. (1993). Volumetric magnetic resonance imaging in men with dementia of the Alzheimer type: correlations with disease severity. *Biol Psychiatry* 34:612–621.

Pantel, J., J. Schroder, and L.R. Schad. (1997). Quantitative magnetic resonance imaging and neuropsychological functions in dementia of the Alzheimer type. *Psychol Med* 27:221–229.

Parnetti, L., D. Lowenthal, and O. Presciutti (1996). ^{1}H-MRS, MRI-based hippocampal volumetry, and ^{99m}Tc-HMPAO-SPECT in normal aging, age-associated memory impairment, and probable Alzheimer's disease from normal aging. *JAGS* 44:133–138.

Pearlson, G.D., G.J. Harris, and R.E. Powers. (1992). Quantitative changes in mesial temporal volume, regional cerebral blood flow, and cognition in Alzheimer's disease. *Arch Gen Psychiatry* 49:402–408.

Petersen, R.C., C.R. Jack, Jr., Y.C. Xu, S.C. Waring, and P.C. O'Brien. (2000). Memory and MRI-based hippocampal volumes in aging and Alzheimer's disease. *Neurology* 54:581–587.

Price, J.L., P.B. Davis, J.C. Morris, and D.L. White. (1991). The distribution of tangles, plaques, and related immunohistochemical markers in healthy aging and Alzheimer's disease. *Neurobiol Aging* 12:295–312.

Rombouts, S., W. Machielsen, M.P. Witter, F. Barkhof, and J. Lindeboom. (1997). Visual association encoding activates the medial temporal lobe: a functional magnetic resonance imaging study. *Hippocampus* 7:594–601.

Rombouts, S., P. Scheltens, W. Machielsen, F. Barkhof, F. Hoogenraad, and D.J. Veltman. (1999). Parametric fMRI analysis of visual encoding in the human medial temporal lobe. *Hippocampus* 9:637–643.

Rusinek, H., M.J. de Leon, and A.E. George. (1991). Alzheimers disease measuring loss of cerebral gray matter with MR imaging. *Radiology* 178:109–114.

Sandson, T.A., O. Felician, R.R. Edelman, and S. Warach. (1999). Diffusion weighted magnetic resonance imaging in Alzheimer's disease. *Dement Geriatr Cogn Disord* 10:166–171.

Scheltens, P., D. Leys, and F. Barkhof. (1992). Atrophy of medial temporal lobes on MRI in "probable" Alzheimer's disease and normal aging: diagnostic value and neuropsychological correlates. *J Neurol Neurosurg Psychiatry* 55:967–972.

Schuff, N., D.L. Amend, and F. Ezekiel. (1997). Changes of hippocampal *N*-acetyl aspartate and volume in Alzheimer's disease: a proton MR spectroscopic imaging and MRI study. *Neurology* 49:1513–1521.

Schuff, N., D.L. Amend, and D.J. Meyerhoff. (1998). Alzheimer's disease: quantitative 1-H MR spectroscopic imaging of frontoparietal brain. *Radiology* 207:91–102.

Seab, J.B., W.J. Jagust, and S.T.S. Wong. (1988). Quantitative NMR measurements of hippocampal atrophy in Alzheimer's disease. *Magn Reson Med* 8:200–208.

Sencakova, D., N.R. Graff-Radford, F.B. Willis, J.A. Lucas, F. Parfitt, R.H. Cha, P.C. O'Brien, R.C. Petersen, and C.R. Jack, Jr. (2001). Hippocampal atrophy correlates with clinical features of Alzheimer's disease in African Americans. *Arch Neurol* 58(10):1593–7.

Shonk, T., and B.D. Ross. (1995a). Role of increased cerebral myo-inositol in the dementia of down syndrome. *MRM* 33:858–861.

Shonk, T.K., R.A. Moats, and P. Gifford. (1995b). Probable Alzheimer disease: diagnosis with proton MR spectroscopy. *Radiology* 195:65–72.

Small, S.A., G.M. Perera, R. DeLaPaz, R. Mayeus, and Y. Stern. (1999). Differential regional dysfunction of the hippocampal formation among elderly with memory decline and Alzheimer's disease. *Ann Neurol* 45: 466–472.

Smith, C.D., A.H. Andersen, R.J. Kryscio, F.A. Schmitt, and M.S. Kindy. (1999a). Altered brain activation in cognitively intact individuals at high risk for Alzheimer's disease. *Neurology* 53:1391–1396.

Smith, C.D., M. Malcein, K. Meurer, F. Schmitt, and W.R. Markesbery. (1999b). MRI temporal lobe volume measures and neuropsychologic function in Alzheimer's disease. *J Neuroimaging* 9:2–9.

Soininen, H.S., K. Partanen, and A. Pitkanen. (1994). Volumetric MRI analysis of the amygdala and the hippocampus in subjects with age-associated memory impairment: correlation to visual and verbal memory. *Neurology* 44:1660–1668.

Stejskal, E.O., and J.E. Tanner. (1965). Spin diffusion measurements: spin-echo in presence of a time dependent field gradient. *J Chem Phys* 42: 288–292.

Stern, C.E., S. Corkin, R.G. Gonzalez, A.R. Guimaraes, and J.R. Baker. (1996). The hippocampal formation participates in novel picture encoding: evidence from functional magnetic resonance imaging. *Proc Natl Acad Sci* 93:8660–8665.

Strange, B.A., P.C. Fletcher, R.N.A. Henson, J.J. Friston, and R.J. Dolan. (1999). Segregating the functions of human hippocampus. *Proc Natl Acad Sci* 96:4034–4039.

Tanabe, J.L., D. Amend, N. Schuff, and V. DiSclafani. (1997). Tissue segmentation of the brain in Alzheimer disease. *AJNR* 18:115–123.

Tedeschi, G., A. Bertolino, and N. Lundbom. (1996). Cortical and subcortical chemical pathology in Alzheimer's disease as assessed by multislice proton magnetic resonance spectroscopic imaging. *Neurology* 47:696–704.

Terry, R.D., A. Peck, and R. DeTeresa. (1981). Some morphometric aspects of the brain in senile dementia of the Alzheimer type. *Ann Neurol* 10: 184–192.

Terry, R.D., E. Masliah, and D.P. Salmon. (1991). Physical basis of cognitive alterations in Alzheimer's disease: synapse loss is the major correlate of cognitive impairment. *Ann Neurol* 30:572–580.

Tomlinson, B.E., G. Blessed, and M. Roth. (1970). Observations on the brains of demented old people. *J Neurol Sci* 11:205–242.

Visser, P.J., P. Scheltens, F.R.J. Verhey, B. Schmand, and L.J. Launer. (1999). Medial temporal lobe atrophy and memory dysfunction as predictors for dementia in subjects with mild cognitive impairment. *J Neurol* 246: 477–485.

Xu, Y., C.R. Jack, Jr., P.C. O'Brien, E. Kokmen, G.E. Smith, R.J. Ivnik, B.F. Boeve, E.G. Tangalos, and R.C. Petersen. (2000). Usefulness of MRI measures of entorhinal cortex vs hippocampus in AD. *Neurology* 54: 1760–1767.

CHAPTER **7**

Functional Imaging

KEITH A. JOHNSON
MARILYN S. ALBERT

Patients with memory complaints are often arrayed along a continuum from normal function through varying degrees of impairment. A crucial question for both patients and clinicians evaluating them is to what extent these complaints are the harbinger of Alzheimer's disease (AD). This issue is of particular importance as strategies for the prevention or delay of dementia are developed. Modern imaging techniques offer one potential method of early detection. In addition, by identifying the neuroimaging measurements useful in the discrimination of prodromal AD, one might learn more about which brain regions are the most affected in the earliest stage of AD. This chapter focuses on the area of functional neuroimaging with radiolabeled tracers, specifically positron emission tomography (PET) and single photon emission computed tomography (SPECT), as they apply to studies of established and prodromal AD.

There is considerable experience with the application of both PET and SPECT to patients with established AD. More recently, these approaches have been expanded to the study of individuals who have a progressive memory difficulty but do not yet meet clinical criteria for AD, or individuals with a genetic risk factor or family history of AD, either with or without a memory problem. Although the findings of these studies are not in uniform agreement, taken together they suggest that a brain network (or networks) with multiple nodes is affected in the earliest stage of AD and that functional imaging techniques, such as PET and SPECT, might facilitate early diagnosis. The nature of these findings is discussed, and their implications for future work are examined.

PERFUSION ABNORMALITIES IN ESTABLISHED ALZHEIMER'S DISEASE

Functional imaging techniques, such as PET and SPECT, have demonstrated specific regional abnormalities in brain perfusion among patients with established AD. The most consistent finding to emerge from these studies is that decreased perfusion or metabolism in the temporoparietal cortex is common among mildly impaired patients with probable AD (e.g., Farkas et al., 1982; Friedland et al., 1983; Foster et al., 1984; Duara et al., 1986; Holman et al., 1992; Johnson et al., 1993). Decreased metabolism has been found in other areas as well, but it is not the predominant pattern reported (McGeer et al., 1990; Smith et al., 1992; Minoshima et al., 1995). Moreover, temporoparietal perfusion abnormalities are increasingly prevalent among patients with moderate and severe AD, leading to increased accuracy of clinical diagnosis based on perfusion data alone (e.g., DeKosky et al., 1990; McGeer et al., 1990; Smith et al., 1992). These abnormalities are also related in a systematic manner to pathological status on autopsy (Jobst et al. 1997).

PERFUSION ALTERATIONS IN PRODROMAL ALZHEIMER'S DISEASE

More recently, investigators have demonstrated brain perfusion alterations among individuals in the prodromal phase of AD. Such studies have been conducted in two types of subject populations: (1) individuals with memory problems who subsequently progressed to the point where they met criteria for AD, and (2) individuals with no cognitive dysfunction but with a genetic mutation known to cause AD.

Regional Perfusion in Late-Onset Prodromal Alzheimer's Disease

To study predictors of the development of late-onset AD, Johnson and colleagues (1998a) obtained SPECT perfusion measures in 80 individuals, about half of whom had evidence of progressive difficulty with memory. This latter group of individuals, whose mean age was 72, did not meet the criteria for AD when the SPECT data were collected. Subsequent evaluations suggest that they were similar in many respects to individuals who meet the criteria for mild cognitive impairment (MCI). As described elsewhere in this volume, MCI is a concept that has recently been introduced to refer to individuals who have memory complaints, normal activities of daily living, and normal general cognitive function but who are memory impaired for their age and are not demented (Petersen et al., 1999). In this SPECT study, all of the controls and the individuals with memory problems were followed annually with a semistructured interview and clinical evaluation to determine which individuals progressed to the point where they met criteria for AD. After 3 years of follow-up, about half of the memory-impaired individuals progressed to AD.

The SPECT data from the baseline evaluation were then examined to determine whether there were SPECT measures that could differentiate the progressers from the normals, and from those individuals who continued to have memory problems but did not progress to the point where they met the criteria for AD. Perfusion abnormalities in four brain regions differentiated the groups: the hippocampal-amygdaloid complex, the posterior cingulate, the anterior thalamus, and the caudal portion of the anterior cingulate. The overall accuracy of discrimination among the groups was 83%. This study also found that perfusion in these four brain regions was abnormal in individuals with established AD, but the most striking abnormalities in cases of established AD were found in the temporoparietal cortex.

A similar study design, using PET, has reported that an alteration in temporoparietal glucose metabolism is also useful in predicting who will develop AD (Arnaiz et al., 2001). These investigators found that glucose metabolism in temporoparietal cortex was decreased in MCI cases who subsequently progressed to AD compared to MCI cases who remained stable (accuracy 75%). Interestingly, another study has reported that decreased temporoparietal metabolism on PET predicts which normal controls will meet criteria for MCI on follow-up (de Leon et al., 2001).

Investigators have also oulined specific regions of interest (ROI), based on a priori hypotheses, to determine whether these targeted measures can predict subsequent development of AD. One SPECT study has reported that the only measure that differentiated controls from prodromal AD cases (accuracy 81%) was decreased perfusion in the posterior cingulate (Okamura et al., 2000). A PET measure of hippocampal metabolism has also been shown to have prognostic value for AD (DeSanti et al., 2001).

Another study has compared the utility of functional vs structural measures for predicting development of AD (i.e., SPECT vs MRI). These investigators (El Fakhri et al., 2001) reported that both methods had similar accuracy in predicting which nondemented individuals with memory problems would progress to AD (82–83% accuracy). Perhaps more importantly, combining the best SPECT and MRI measures yielded systematically better results than using either MRI or SPECT data alone. This suggests that different information is present in the SPECT and MRI data which can help predict who will develop AD over time.

Regional Perfusion in Early-Onset Prodromal Alzheimer's Disease

SPECT has also been used to examine individuals who are in the prodromal phase of AD by virtue of the presence of a genetic mutation. The majority of patients with Alzheimer's disease who are under the age of 60 carry a mutation in the presenilin-1 (*PS-1*) gene. At least 50 such mutations on the *PS-1* gene have been identified among over 80 families of various ethnic origins (Cruts et al., 1998). These mutations confer autosomal dominant inheritance, with virtually 100% penetrance. One of these mutations, which occurs at codon 280 in the *PS-1* gene, has been identified in a large multigenerational family living in Colombia, South America (Lopera et al., 1997). The average age of onset of AD in this kindred is 47 years. Individuals with this mutation will therefore eventually develop AD, if they live through the age of risk, whether or not they are symptomatic at any one point in time.

A SPECT study has been conducted comparing asymptomatic individuals who carried a *PS-1* mutation, to individuals with the mutation who had AD, and to individuals who did not carry the *PS-1* mutation and were cognitively normal from the same multigenerational family (Johnson et al., 1998b, 2001). This study found that subjects with the *PS-1* mutation who were asymptomatic demonstrated less perfusion than did the normal controls in the hippocampal complex, the anterior and posterior cingulate, the posterior parietal lobe, and the anterior frontal lobe. The AD patients demonstrated less perfusion in the posterior parietal and superior frontal cortex than did the normal controls. Using these SPECT measures, 86% of these groups of subjects could be accurately differentiated from one another.

Kennedy et al. (1995) used PET to evaluate asymptomatic individuals from families with another autosomal dominant form of AD. They demonstrated lower glucose metabolism in temporoparietal cortical regions among such subjects. Thus, both SPECT and PET have demonstrated that regional cerebral perfusion abnormalities are detectable before the clinical symptoms of AD develop in carriers of the *PS-1* mutation.

PERFUSION ALTERATIONS IN *APOE-4* CARRIERS

Several studies of cerebral perfusion have also been conducted in subjects with the one widely agreed on genetic risk factor for late-onset AD: the *E4* allele of the apolipoprotein E (*APOE*) gene. The *E4* allele of the *APOE* gene is associated with an increased risk for AD and modifies age of onset (Saunders et al. 1993). For example, an individual with no copies of the *E4* allele has a lifetime risk of developing AD of 9%, whereas the presence of one *E4* allele increases lifetime risk for AD to 29% (Swartz et al., 1999). However, the *E4* allele does not act as a dominant, fully penetrant gene. Thus, many subjects who have two copies of the *E4* allele never develop AD, and approximately one-half of the people who develop AD have no copies of the *E4* allele.

Regional Perfusion in *E4* Carriers Who Do Not Meet Criteria for Alzheimer's Disease

There is considerable agreement that individuals who do not meet criteria for AD have *E4*-associated decreases in cerebral perfusion. Small et al. (1995) examined subjects with mild memory problems who were *E4* positive and had a family history of AD. Using PET, they found decreased parietal metabolism in the *E4* carriers (other regions of the brain were not examined). Subsequently, Reiman and colleagues (1996), also using PET, examined subjects who were homozygous for the *E4* allele but did not demonstrate evidence of memory problems. This group of asymptomatic at-risk subjects demonstrated decreased metabolism in temporoparietal cortical regions. The investigators also found perfusion decreases in the posterior cingulate and prefrontal cortex.

These findings have been confirmed and extended by a recent study in which nondemented *E4* carriers with memory problems demonstrated lower glucose metabolism in the inferior parietal lobe, the lateral temporal cortex, and the posterior cingulate (Small et al., 2000). In addition, lower glucose metabolism at baseline predicted declines in memory performance 2 years later, although the *E4* group as a whole did not demonstrate a significant decline in memory over that interval, as compared with individuals who did not have an *E4* allele.

Reiman and colleagues (2001) reported a similar finding with a group of individuals who had a family history of AD and were also heterozygous for the APOE-4 allele. They found decreases in the temporal, posterior cingulate, and prefrontal cortex, as well as in the basal forebrain, the parahippocampal gyrus, and the thalamus (Reiman et al., 2001).

It remains unknown, however, how many of the individuals with decreases in glucose metabolism will develop AD over time. To date, few subjects in either of these cohorts have progressed to this point.

Regional Perfusion in *E4* Carriers with Alzheimer's Disease

Studies of individuals with AD, both with and without the *E4* allele, have also been conducted. These have produced contradictory findings, however. The investigations have used both PET and SPECT to determine whether there is a perfusion pattern that is characteristic of the *APOE-4* genotype in AD patients, unrelated to their disease status (Corder et al., 1997; Higuchi et al.,

1997; Lehtovirta et al., 1998; Sperling et al., 1998; VanDyck et al., 1998). Some studies have found no distinct perfusion pattern (e.g., Corder et al., 1997; Hirono et al., 1998), while others have reported decreases in cortical perfusion or asymmetries in cortical perfusion that vary considerably from study to study (e.g., Lehtovirta et al., 1998; Sperling et al., 1998; VanDyck et al., 1998). One longitudinal study reported significant declines in occipital perfusion among AD patients carrying an *E4* allele but no relationship between the declines in functional severity and perfusion over the 3 year interval (Lehtovirta et al., 1998).

BRAIN NETWORKS IMPLICATED IN PRODROMAL ALZHEIMER'S DISEASE

Despite the variety of functional imaging studies conducted to date, the findings suggest that a consistent set of brain regions are affected in prodromal AD. These regions include the hippocampal complex, the anterior and posterior cingulate, and the inferior parietal cortex.

Hippocampal Formation

Perfusion alterations in the hippocampal complex in prodromal AD are consistent with a large body of knowledge indicating that this region is involved at the earliest stage of this disorder (e.g., Ball, 1977; Hyman et al., 1984; Gómez-Isla et al., 1996). Recent neuropathological studies indicate that the pathological hallmarks of AD (i.e., the neurofibrillary tangles and neuritic plaques) are first evident in the entorhinal cortex (Gómez-Isla et al., 1996). This finding is consistent with the fact that most patients with AD have a progressive memory impairment as their earliest cognitive problem (Moss et al., 1986; Welsh et al., 1992). The entorhinal cortex is a portion of the anterior parahippocampal gyrus that gives rise to the perforant pathway, the major cortical excitatory input to the hippocampus, and receives projections from widespread limbic and association areas. As such, it is part of a memory-related neural system in the brain (Zola et al., 2000).

Anterior and Posterior Cingulate

The perfusion alterations found in the posterior cingulate and the anterior thalamus in prodromal AD, and in those at risk for the disease because of family history or genetic profile, are also consistent with the fact that a striking memory impairment is seen in the earliest stage of AD. Recent studies in rodents indicate that the hippocampal formation and the posterior cingulate (together with the anterior thalamus) make up a memory system that is critical for learning the relationships among cues, such as previously unrelated spatial or temporal features of the environment (Sutherland and Rudy, 1989, 1991). Neuroanatomic studies in monkeys also demonstrate strong interconnections between these three brain regions (Pandya and Seltzer, 1982; Vogt et al., 1987; Van Hoesen et al., 1991). It should be noted that perfusion abnormalities in the posterior cingulate have also been described in established AD (Minoshima et al., 1994).

The perfusion abnormalities found in the caudal portion of the anterior cingulate and the prefrontal cortex during prodromal AD, and in those at risk for the disease, are consistent with evidence that executive function (e.g., set shifting, self-monitoring) deficits are prevalent in patients with very mild AD (Lafleche and Albert, 1995), and among patients in the prodromal phase of the disease (Albert et al., 2001). The caudal portion of the anterior cingulate is strongly and reciprocally connected with the prefrontal cortex. It is also strongly and reciprocally connected with memory-related structures, including the entorhinal cortex (Vogt et al., 1991; Van Hoesen and Solodkin, 1993). Thus, it has been hypothesized that the caudal portion of the anterior cingulate plays a major role in executive function abilities, primarily through its reciprocal connections with the prefrontal cortex (Arikuni et al., 1994).

Inferior Parietal Cortex

The perfusion abnormalities found in the inferior parietal cortex in individuals at risk for AD are consistent with the fact that temporoparietal perfusion defects are common in established AD, as described here. However, their relationship to the symptoms of individuals in the prodromal phase of AD are less clear, since abnormalities in temporoparietal cortices have not been associated with either memory or executive function deficits. Likewise, the neuropathological changes associated with AD have not been reported to affect this cortical area at the earliest stage of AD. It has therefore been hypothesized that perfusion abnormalities are evident in temporoparietal cortices because they contain distal projections of dendritic fields from the hippocampal complex (Meguro et al., 1999). In this context, it should be noted that temporoparietal changes among individuals at risk for AD have only been shown in studies that performed PET scanning, and thus methodological characteristics unique to PET may be responsible for this result. Moreover, the data regarding perfusion patterns related to *APOE-4* genotype alone have been contradictory. Therefore it has been difficult to determine with any certainty when in the course of disease, temporal or parietal cortical perfusion abnormalities begin to predominate.

IMPLICATIONS OF FUNCTIONAL IMAGING IN PRODROMAL ALZHEIMER'S DISEASE

The functional imaging findings in prodromal AD just described are of considerable theoretical interest. They indicate that there are alterations in a distributed brain network (or networks) in prodromal AD, which are measurable with functional neuroimaging. They confirm previous hypotheses about the importance of temporoparietal cortical abnormalities in full-blown AD. More important, they suggest that a set of brain structures show selective changes before the time that individuals meet the criteria for AD, including changes in the anterior and posterior cingulate and the hippocampal complex. Thus, additional hypotheses have been generated by these functional imaging data concerning the brain regions that are involved in prodromal AD and their potential effect on cognitive decline.

These findings also have potential clinical significance, since, in theory, measures of perfusion or metabolism could be used to identify individuals in the prodromal phase of AD for clinical intervention. The highest accuracy of identification that has been reported to date is approximately 85%. If a proposed treatment were relatively benign, one could consider using a functional imaging method with this degree of accuracy to enrich a sample of individuals who were likely to develop AD within a few years. However, if the potential treatment produced significant side effects, which appears likely, then a higher level of accuracy would be needed. This suggests that functional imaging procedures would need to be combined with other information about the subjects, such as their cognitive performance, in order to achieve the accuracy needed to identify high-risk individuals for treatment trials.

A greater understanding of the clinical characteristics of subjects with MCI is also needed to fully exploit the use of functional imaging as a potential marker of early AD. For example, it is not yet known whether the findings described in this chapter can be generalized to the entire at-risk population, since the studies reported here have been based on groups of research subjects who were carefully selected to eliminate confounding conditions and then followed over time. It is known that, even in such selected populations, not everyone with subtle memory difficulties progresses to develop AD within a few years (e.g., Daly et al., 2000).

Moreover, differences in the populations that have been selected for study add to this variability in outcome. For example, after an average follow-up of 2 years, the rates of progression to AD reported in the literature vary between 80% and 24% (Rubin et al., 1989; Flicker et al., 1991; Petersen et al., 1994; Devanand et al., 1997; Tierney et al., 1996). This variability could be occurring for several reasons: (*1*) the group of individuals with evidence of recent and progressive difficulties in memory may be heterogeneous in nature; (*2*) the characteristics of the populations under study may be based on different selection criteria; and (*3*) the criteria for progression to AD may be applied in different ways.

Recent findings suggest that the first two explanations are almost certainly correct (Daly et al., 2000), thus emphasizing the importance of comparing the selection methods used by different research groups. For example, it is already evident that memory-impaired individuals who have been studied in the prodromal phase of AD do not, in all cases, meet criteria for MCI. All subjects with prodromal AD tend to be similar to subjects with MCI in that they have memory complaints, normal activities of daily living, and normal general cognitive function, and they are memory impaired for their age but are not demented. However, it is typical for individuals with MCI to score 1.5 SD below the mean of their peer group on tests of memory, and, in fact, some research studies use this range of performance as one of the selection criteria for MCI (Petersen, 2000). However, some investigators have studied individuals with prodromal AD who appear to have lower levels of cognitive impairment than is typical of individuals with MCI (e.g., Johnson et al., 1998), suggesting at least one source for the variability in crossover rates among studies. This may also contribute to differences in the findings from functional imaging.

It should also be noted that there are differences in the crossover rate among the controls in the ongoing studies of prodromal AD, adding further sources of variability. Some studies report that 1% to 2% of their controls "convert" to AD on a yearly basis (e.g., Petersen et al., 1998a), while others report no conversions to AD among controls after more than 3 years of follow-up (Daly et al., 2000). It will be important to learn more about the factors that influence the rate of progression or stability among individuals with and without progressive memory problems in order to generalize the functional imaging findings described here to the population as a whole.

Additional work is also needed to identify the source of the discrepancies among studies that have examined the pattern of perfusion associated with the *APOE-4* genotype. The contradictory nature of these findings makes it difficult to determine whether the perfusion patterns seen among individuals who are at risk for AD differ in substantive ways from those based on genotype alone. This is particularly important since the *E4* allele increases risk for atherosclerosis as well as AD, and there remains the possibility that PET and SPECT are sensitive to such factors associated with the *APOE-4* genotype, rather than being predictive of AD.

Thus, much work remains to be done, including the replication of these initial, promising studies; the refinement of functional imaging techniques by registration with underlying structural images; the inclusion of a subject mix that is representative of those at risk for AD, and further studies examining the effect of the *APOE-4* genotype alone on regional cerebral perfusion.

Acknowledgments

The preparation of this manuscript was supported by grant no. PO1-AG04953 from the National Institute on Aging.

References

Albert, M., M. Moss, R. Tanzi, and K. Jones. (2001). Preclinical prediction of AD using neuropsychological tests. *J Intnatl Neuropsych Soc* 7:631–639.

Arikuni, T., H. Sako, and A. Murata. (1994). Ipsilateral connections of the anterior cingulate cortex with the frontal and medial temporal cortices in the macaque monkey. *Neurosci Res* 21:19–39.

Arnaiz, E., V. Jelic, O. Almkvist, L. Wahlund, B. Winblad, S. Valind, and A. Nordberg. (2001). Impaired glucose metabolism and cognitive functioning predict deterioration in mild cognitive impairment. *Neuroreport* 12:851–855.

Ball, M.J. (1977). Neuronal loss, neurofibrillary tangles and granulovacuolar degeneration in the hippocampus with ageing and dementia: a quantitative study. *Acta Neuropathol* 37:111–118.

Corder, E., V. Jelic, H. Basun, et al. (1997). No difference in cerebral glucose metabolism in patients with Alzheimer's disease and differing apolipoprotern E genotypes. *Arch Neurol* 54:273–277.

Cruts, M., C. van Duijn, H. Backhovens, M. Van den Broeck, A. Wehnert, S. Serneels, R. Sherrington, M. Hutton, J. Hardy, P. St. George-Hyslop, A. Hofman, and C. Van Broeckhoven. (1998). Estimation of the genetic contribution of presenilin 1 and 2 mutations in a population-based study of presenilin Alzheimer disease. *Hum Mol Genet* 7:43–51.

Daly, B., D. Zaitchik, M. Copeland, J. Schmahmann, J. Gunther, and M. Albert. (2000). Predicting "conversion" to AD using standardized clinical information. *Arch Neurol* 57:675–680.

DeKosky, S., W-J. Shih, F. Schmitt, J. Coupal, and C. Kirkpatrick. (1990). Assessing utility of single photon emission computed tomography (SPECT) scan in Alzheimer disease: correlation with cognitive severity. *Alzheimer Dis Assoc Disorders* 4:14–23.

de Leon, M., A. Convit, O. Wolf, C. Tarshish, S. DeSanti, M. Rusinek, W. Tsui, E. Kandil, A. Scherer, A. Roche, A. Imossi, E. Thorn, M. Bobinski, C. Caraos, P. Lesbre, D. Schyler, J. Poirier, and B. Reisberg. (2001). Prediction of cognitive decline in normal elderly subjects with 2-[^{18}Fluoro-2-deoxy-d-glucose/positron emission tomography (FDG/PET). *Proc Natl Acad Sci* 98:10966–10977.

DeSanti, S., M. deLeon, H. Rusinek, A. Convit, C. Tarshish, A. Roche, W. Tsui, E. Kandil, M. Boppana, K. Daisley, G. Wang, D. Schlyer, and J. Fowler. (2001). Hippocampal formation glucose metabolism and volume losses in MCI and AD. *Neurobiol Aging,* 22:529–539.

Devanand, D., M. Felz, M. Gorlyn, J. Moeller, and Y. Stern. (1997). Questionable dementia: clinical course and predictors of outcome. *J Am Geriatr Soc* 45:321–328.

Duara, R., C. Grady, J. Haxby, M. Sundaram, N.R. Cutler, L. Heston, A. Moore, N. Schlageter, S. Larson, and S.I. Rapoport. (1986). Positron emission tomography in Alzheimer's disease. *Neurology* 36:879–887.

El Fakrhi, G., M. Kijewski, J. Hilson, K. Johnson, R. Zimmerman, A. Becker, R. Killiany, K. Jones, and M. Albert. (2001). Quantitative SPECT and volumetric MRI for discimination between normal controls and pre-clinical Alzheimer's disease. *Eur J Nucl Med* 8:1059.

Farkas, T., S.H. Ferris, A.P. Wolf, M.J. De Leon, D.R. Christman, B. Reisberg, A. Alavi, J.S. Fowler, A.E. George, and M. Reivich. (1982). 18F-2-deoxy-2-fluoro-D-glucose as a tracer in the positron emission tomographic study of senile dementia. *Am J Psychiatry* 139:352–353.

Flicker, C., S. Ferris, and B. Reisberg. (1991). Mild cognitive impairment in the elderly: predictors of dementia. *Neurology* 41:1006–1009.

Foster, N.L., T.N. Chase, L. Mansi, R. Brooks, P. Fedio, N.J. Patronas, and G. Di Chiro. (1984). Cortical abnormalities in Alzheimer's disease. *Ann Neurol* 16:649–654.

Friedland, R.H., T.F. Budinger, E. Ganz, Y. Yano, C.A. Mathis, B. Koss, B.A. Ober, R.H. Huesman, and S.E. Derenzo. (1983). Regional cerebral metabolic alterations in dementia of the Alzheimer type: positron emission tomography with [18F]fluorodeoxyglucose. *J Comput Assist Tomogr* 7: 590–598.

Gómez-Isla, T., J.L. Price, D.W. McKeel Jr, J.C. Morris, J.H. Growdon, and B.T. Hyman. (1996). Profound loss of layer II entorhinal cortex neurons occurs in very mild Alzheimer's disease. *J Neurosci* 16:4491–4500.

Gómez-Isla, T., R. Hollister, H. West, S. Mui, J.H. Growdon, R.C. Petersen, J.E. Parisi, and B.T. Hyman. (1997). Neuronal loss correlates with but exceeds neurofibrillary tangles in Alzheimer's disease. *Ann Neurol* 41: 17–24.

Higuchi, M., H. Arai, T. Nakagawa, S. Higuchi, T. Muramatsu, S. Matsushita, Y. Kosaka, M. Itoh, and H. Sasaki. (1997). Regional cerebral glucose utilization is modulated by the dosage of apolipoprotein E type 4 allele and alpha1-antichymotrypsin type A allele in Alzheimer's disease. *Neuroreport* 8:2639–2643.

Hirono, N., E. Mori, M. Yasuda, et al. (1998). Lack of association of apolipoprotein E E4 allele dose with cerebral glucose metabolism in Alzheimer disease. *Alzheimer Dis Assoc Disord* 12:362–367.

Holman, B.L., K.A. Johnson, B. Gerada, P.A. Carvalho, and A. Satlin. (1992). The scintigraphic appearance of Alzheimer's disease: a prospective study using technetium-99m-HMPAO SPECT. *J Nucl Med* 33: 181–185.

Hyman, B.T., G.W. Van Horsen, A.R. Damasio, and Barnes C.L. (1984). Alzheimer's disease: cell-specific pathology isolates the hippocampal formation. *Science* 225:1168–1170.

Jobst, K., L. Barneston, and B. Shepstone. (1997). Accurate prediction of histologically confirmed Alzheimer's disease and the differential diagnosis of dementia: the use of NINCDS-ADRDA and DSM III-R criteria, SPECT, x-ray CT and APOE4 medial temporal lobe dementias. *Int Psychogeriatr* 9:191–222.

Johnson, K.A., M.F. Kijewski, J.A. Becker, B. Garada, A. Satlin, and B.L. Holman. (1993). Quantitative brain SPECT in Alzheimer's disease and normal aging. *J Nucl Med* 34:2044–2048.

Johnson, K.A., K.J. Jones, J.A. Becker, A. Satlin, B.L. Holman, and M.S. Albert. (1998a). Preclinical prediction of Alzheimer's disease using SPECT. *Neurology* 50:1563–1571.

Johnson, K., F. Lopera, K. Jones, A. Becker, R. Sperling, J. Hilson, J. Londono, I. Siegert, M. Arcos, S. Moreno, L. Madrigal, J. Ossa, N. Pineda, A. Ardila, M. Roselli, M. Albert, K. Kosik, and A. Rios. (2001). Presenilin-1-associated abnormalities in regional cerebral perfusion. *Neurology* 56:1545–1551.

Kennedy, A.M., R.S. Frackowiak, S.K. Newman, P.M. Bloomfield, J. Seaward, P. Roques, G. Lewington, V.J. Cunningham, and M.N. Rossor. (1995). Deficits in cerebral glucose metabolism demonstrated by positron emission tomography in individuals at risk of familial Alzheimer's disease. *Neurosci Lett* 186:17–20.

Lafleche, G., and M. Albert. (1995). Executive function deficits in mild Alzheimer's disease. *Neuropsychology* 9:313–320.

Lehtovirta, M., J. Kuikka, S. Helisalmi, P. Hartikainen, A. Mannermaa, M. Ryynanen, P. Riekkinen Sr, and H. Soininen. (1998). Longitudinal SPECT study in Alzheimer's disease: relation to apolipoprotein E polymorphism. *J Neurol Neurosurg Psychiatry* 64:742–746.

Lopera, F., A. Ardilla, A. Martinez, L. Madrigal, J. Arango-Viana, C. Lemere, J. Arango-Lasprilla, L. Hincapie, M. Arcos-Burgos, J. Ossa, I. Behrens, J. Norton, C. Lendon, A. Goate, A. Ruiz-Linares, M. Roselli, and K. Kosik. (1997). Clinical features of early-onset Alzheimer disease in a large kindred with an E280A presenilin-1 mutation. *JAMA* 277:793–799.

McGeer, E.G., P.L. McGeer, R. Harrop, H. Akiyama, and H. Kamo. (1990). Correlations of regional postmortem enzyme activities with premortem local glucose metabolic rates in Alzheimer's disease. *J Neurosci Res* 27:612–619.

Meguro, K., X. Blaizot, Y. Kondoh, C. LeMestric, J. Baron, and C. Chavoix. (1999). Neocortical and hippocampal glucose metabolism following neurotoxic lesions of the entorhinal and perirhinal cortices in the nonhuman primate. *Brain* 2:1519–1531.

Minoshima, S., N.L. Foster, and D.E. Kuhl. (1994). Posterior cingulate cortex in Alzheimer's disease [letter]. *Lancet* 344:895.

Minoshima, S., K. Frey, R. Koeppe, N. Foster, and D. Kuhl. (1995). A diagnostic approach to Alzheimer's disease using three-dimensional stereotactic surface projections of fluorine-18-FDG PET. *J Nucl Med* 36:1238–1248.

Moss, M.B., M.S. Albert, N. Butters, and M. Payne. (1986). Differential patterns of memory loss among patients with Alzheimer's disease, Huntington's disease, and alcoholic Korsakoff's syndrome. *Arch Neurol* 43:239–246.

Okamura, N., M. Shinkawa, H. Arai, T. Matsui, K. Nakajo, M. Maruyama, X. Hu, and H. Sasaki. (2000). Prediction of progression of patients with mild cognitive impairment using IMP-SPECT. *Nippon Ronen Igakkai Zasshi* 37:974–978.

Pandya, D.N., and B. Seltzer. (1982). Intrinsic connections and architectonics of posterior parietal cortex in the rhesus monkey. *Comp Neurol* 204:196–210.

Petersen, R. (2000). Mild cognitive impairment or questionable dementia? *Arch Neurol* 57:643–644.

Petersen, R., G. Smith, R. Ivnik, E. Kokmen, and E. Tangalos. (1994). Memory function in very early Alzheimer's disease. *Neurology* 44:867–872.

Petersen, R., G. Smith, S. Waring, R. Ivnik, E. Tangalos, and E. Kokmen. (1999). Mild cognitive impairment: clinical characterization and outcome. *Arch Neurol* 56:303–308.

Reiman, E., R. Caselli, K. Chen, G. Alexander, D. Bandy, and J. Frost. (2001). Declining brain activity in cognitively normal apolipoprotein E varepsilon heterozygotes: A foundation for using positron emission tomography to efficiently test treatments to prevent Alzheimer's disease. *Proc Natl Acad Sci* 98:3334–3339.

Reiman, E.M., R.J. Caselli, L.S. Yun, K. Chen, D. Bandy, S. Minoshima, S.N. Thibodeau, and D. Osborne. (1996). Preclinical evidence of Alzheimer's disease in persons homozygous for the epsilon 4 allele for apolipoprotein E. *N Engl J Med* 334:752–758.

Rubin, E., J. Morris, E. Grant, and T. Vendegna. (1989). Very mild senile dementia of the Alzheimer's type. I: Clinical assessment. *Arch Neurol* 46:379–382.

Saunders, A.M., O. Hulette, K.A. Welsh-Bohmer, D.E. Schmechel, B. Crain, J.R. Burke, M.J. Alberts, W.J. Strittmatter, J.C. Breitner, and C. Rosenberg. (1993). Specificity, sensitivity, and predictive value of apolipoprotein-E genotyping for sporadic Alzheimer's disease. *Lancet* 348: 90–93.

Small, G.W., J.C. Mazziotta, M.T. Collins, L.R. Baxter, M.E. Phelps, M.A. Mandelkern, A. Kaplan, A. La Rue, C.F. Adamson, L. Chang et al. (1995). Apolipoprotein E type 4 allele and cerebral glucose metabolism in relatives at risk for familial Alzheimer disease. *JAMA* 273:942–947.

Small, G., L. Ercoli, D. Silverman, S.-C. Huang, S. Komo, S. Bookheimer, H. Lawretsky, K. Miller, R. Siddarth, N. Rasgon, J. Mazziotta, S. Saxena, H. Wu, M. Megal, J. Cummings, A. Saunders, M. Pericak-Vance, A. Roses, J. Barrio, and M. Phelps. (2000). Cerebral metabolic and cognitive decline in persons at genetic risk for Alzheimer's disease. *PNAS* 97:6037–6042.

Smith, G.S., M.J. de Leon, A.E. George, A. Kluger, N.D. Volkow, T. McRae, J. Golomb, S.H. Ferris, B. Reisberg, J. Ciaravino, et al. (1992). Topography of cross-sectional and longitudinal glucose metabolic deficits in Alzheimer's disease: pathophysiologic implications. *Arch Neurol* 49: 1142–1150.

Sperling, R., K. Jones, D. Rentz, M. Albert, L. Holman, J. Becker, L. Scinto, K. Daffner, and K. Johnson. (1998). SPECT cerebral perfusion and apolipoprotein E genotype. *Neurology* 58:S70.

Sutherland, R.J., and J.W. Rudy. (1989). Configurational association theory: the role of the hippocampal formation in learning, memory and amnesia. *Psychobiology* 17:129–144.

Sutherland, R.J., and J.W. Rudy. (1991). Exceptions to the rule of space. *Hippocampus* 1:250–252.

Swartz, R., S. Black, and P. St. George-Hyslop. (1999). Apolipoprotein E and Alzheimer's disease: a genetic, molecular and neuroimaging review. *Canad J Neurol Sci* 26:77–88.

Tierney, M., J. Szalai, W. Snow, R. Fisher, A. Nores, G. Nadon, E. Dunn, and P. St. George-Hyslop. (1996). Prediction of probable Alzheimer's disease in memory impaired patients: a prospective longitudinal study. *Neurology* 46:661–665.

VanDyck, C., J. Gelernter, M. MacAvoy, R. Avery, M. Criden, O. Okereke, P. Varma, J. Seibyl, and P. Hoffer. (1998). Absence of an apolipoprotein E ε4 allele associated with increased parietal regional cerebral blood flow asymmetry in Alzheimer disease. *Arch Neurol* 55:1460–1466.

Van Hoesen, G.W., and A. Solodkin. (1993). Some modular features of temporal cortex in humans as revealed by pathological changes in Alzheimer's disease. *Cereb Cortex* 3:465–475.

Van Hoesen, G.W., B.T. Hyman, and A.R. Damasio. (1991). Entorhinal cortex pathology in Alzheimer's disease. *Hippocampus* 1:1–8.

Vogt, B.A., D.N. Pandya, and D.L. Rosene. (1987). Cingulate cortex of the rhesus monkey. I: Cytoarchitecture and thalamic afferents. *J Comp Neurol* 262:256–270.

Vogt, B.A., P.B. Crino, and L. Volicer. (1991). Laminar alterations in γ-aminobutyric acid A, muscarinic, and β adrenoceptors and neuron degeneration in cingulate cortex in Alzheimer's disease. *J Neurochem* 57: 282–290.

Welsh, K.A., N. Butters, J.P. Hughes, R.C. Mohs, and A. Heyman. (1992). Detection and staging of dementia in Alzheimer's disease: use of the neuropsychological measures developed for the Consortium to Establish a Registry for Alzheimer's Disease. *Arch Neurol* 49:448–452.

Zola, S., L. Squire, E. Teng, L. Stefanacci, E. Bufallo, and R. Clark. (2000). Impaired recognition memory in monkeys after damage limited to the hippocampal region. *J Neurosci* 20:451–463.

CHAPTER **8**

Spectrum of Pathology

HEIKO BRAAK
KELLY DEL TREDICI
EVA BRAAK

In recent decades, the population of developed industrial countries has experienced a marked prolongation of life expectancy. The distressing aspect of this advance is an alarming increase in the prevalence of age-associated degenerative brain diseases. The etiologies of many of these illnesses are still unknown. Study of these diseases requires detailed knowledge of age-related brain alterations in order to permit a clear differentiation of the lesions related to disease.

Phases of brain aging often are viewed somewhat naively as "normal" stages of the life cycle comparable to the phases of brain development and maturation. Nonetheless, it should be taken into account that phases of human brain aging generally are not foreseen in nature's plan and are rendered possible only under favorable conditions. Subhuman mammals and humans living under harsh natural conditions typically attain only a fraction of their potential life expectancies. For the last several thousand years, civilization has provided a protective framework that artificially enables some human beings to survive long enough for age-associated brain changes to become apparent.

The brain has almost nothing in common with a computer or a technical device. Nearly all of the nerve cells constituting the human brain are postmitotic elements and attain approximately the same age as the individual to whom they belong. This does not imply, however, that they remain a static network of cells with countless immutable connections. On the contrary, the structure of nerve cells is modified continuously, not only during early development but also during the apparently stable phase of maturity and—what is more easily detectable—in senescence. Contrary to popular belief, it is not at all clear whether all of the morphological changes occurring in early development truly represent progressive refinement or whether all of the alterations appearing in old age are classifiable as decrements in the complexity of the brain. Progressive alterations, such as growth and refinement of neuronal processes, and regressive changes probably take place simultaneously and even at the same locations. The living brain continuously undergoes subtle structural permutations. The response to the aging process varies greatly among different types of nerve cells, as well as among different types of glial cells and nonneuroectodermal cells.

The morphological alterations related to Alzheimer's disease (AD) develop in only a few susceptible neuronal types. The lesions initially evolve at predisposed cortical induction sites, whence they encroach in a predictable, nonrandom manner on other territories of the brain. A continuum exists from the first lesion to the far-reaching destruction seen in fully developed AD. No single feature permits definition of a specific form of AD-related pathological changes that is exclusively related to aging. Accordingly, the lesions should not be viewed as normal concomitants of aging, although they become increasingly prevalent with age (Braak and Braak, 1997; Hyman and Trojanowski, 1997; Hyman and Gómez-Isla, 1998; Green et al., 2000).

Availability of an adequate animal model would greatly foster the study of age- and disease-related morphological changes in the human brain (Schultz et al., 2000a, 2000b). Although small rodents are indispensable to geriatric research because their life spans are short and they are easily manipulated genetically (Brion et al., 1999; Seabrook and Rosahl, 1999; Götz, 2001; Janus and Westaway, 2001), the murine cerebral cortex differs considerably from that of humans. It lacks the specific neuronal types, cortical areas, and layers that characterize the human brain. Whereas age-related changes in the human brain typically are encountered in neocortical layers IIIa and IIIb, these layers are missing in the murine brain or are present only in a preliminary developmental stage. As such, aging in the human brain and the outcome of many neurodegenerative diseases cannot be adequately understood by extrapolating data from transgenic mice or other species of experimental animal. Investigations of the human brain are, and will remain, irreplaceable in the endeavor to comprehend both disease-related destruction and age-associated improvements or impairments in human brain function.

ANATOMICAL BACKGROUND

Constituents of the Cerebral Cortex

The preeminent directive entity of the human central nervous system is the cerebral cortex. Its neuronal constituents are composed of many types of pyramidal neurons and a heterogeneous group of nonpyramidal nerve cells (Braak, 1980; Feldman, 1984; Zilles, 1990; Nieuwenhuys, 1994). Pyramidal neurons and modified pyramidal cells occur in all cortical cellular layers and areas. Most generate an axon that enters the white matter and terminates in other areas or subcortical nuclei. The nonpyramidal cells (local circuit neurons), by contrast, generate an axon that branches profusely in the vicinity of the parent soma. The axon of pyramidal neurons and frequently also its collateral branches become myelinated distal to the initial segment. Functional maturity of these cells is achieved only after myelination of the axon and establishment of bidirectional synaptic contacts to local circuit neurons. Projection cells, oligodendroglial cells maintaining the myelin sheath of axons, and local circuit neurons thus work together to form the essential components of a functional cortical unit.

The cortex displays a variable content of myelinated fibers. Radiant bundles consist of fibers perpendicular to the surface, whereas myelinated lines run parallel to it. The inner and outer lines of Baillarger, located in neocortical layers IV and Vb, consist chiefly of myelinated axon collaterals of pyramidal cells. Sublayers IIIa and IIIb show a tendency to separate from IIIc, fore-shadowing a future increase in the number of neocortical layers. The affiliated myelinated plexus is the late-maturing line of Kaes Bechterew in IIIb, which can be recognized in only a few neo-cortical areas.

The brain of the human adult is exceptionally richly sup-plied with intraneuronal deposits of lipofuscin or neuromelanin and differs remarkably in this respect from the brain of subhu-man primates. The cell bodies of cortical pyramidal neurons usu-ally contain small, evenly distributed lipofuscin granules, whereas nonpyramidal cells are either free of such pigment or densely filled with it. Many neuronal types display a modest increment in the number of lipofuscin granules with age, but this does not affect the pigmentation differences between pyramidal cells and nonpyramidal cells (Braak, 1980, 1984).

Subdivisions of the Cerebral Cortex

Recognition of major age changes and AD-related lesions is fa-cilitated by introducing simplified diagrams of the interconnec-tions between important cortical areas and a few subcortical nu-clei (Figs. 8–1, 8–2). The telencephalic cortex is not a uniform entity; rather, it consists of two different types of gray matter: the neocortex and the allocortex. The allocortex is confined largely to the anteromedial portions of the temporal lobe and includes limbic system centers such as the hippocampal formation and the entorhinal region. The subcortical nuclear complex of the amygdala is closely related to these. The parietal, occipital, and temporal neocortices each consist of a primary field (core), flanked by a belt of unimodal first order association areas, which, in turn, is accompanied by far-reaching unimodal or heteromo-dal high order sensory association areas (Braak, 1980; Zilles, 1990).

Visual, somatosensory, and auditory data proceed through the neocortical primary sensory fields and adjoining first order sensory association areas to the related high order sensory as-sociation areas and then are conveyed via long corticocortical projections to the prefrontal cortical areas (Fig. 8–1). Tracts gen-erated in this highest organizational level of the brain conduct the data through the premotor areas (belt) to the primary motor field (core). The striatal and cerebellar loops, however, provide

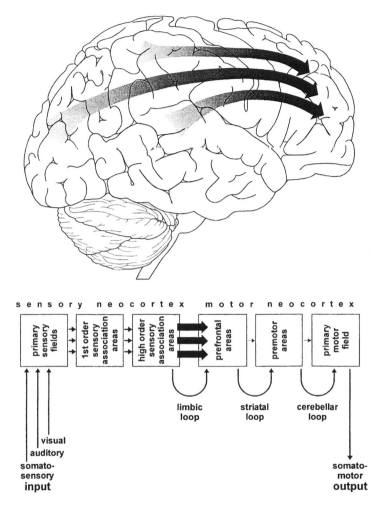

Figure 8–1. Visual, somatosensory, and auditory information proceeds through the respective neocortical primary sensory fields and first-order sensory association areas to a variety of high order sensory association areas; then the data are transported via long corticocortical pathways to the prefrontal areas. Tracts generated from this highest organizational level of the brain guide the data back via the premotor areas to the primary motor field. The striatal and cerebellar loops provide the major routes for this transport from the prefrontal areas to the primary motor field.

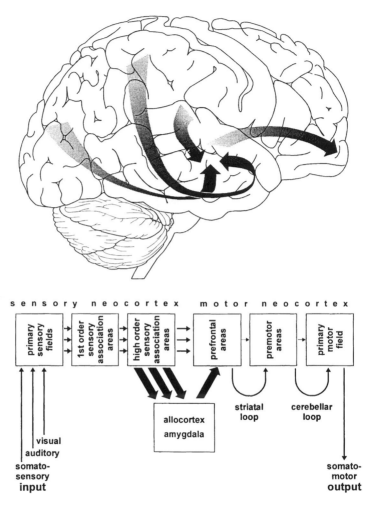

Figure 8–2. Part of the stream of data from the high order sensory association areas to the prefrontal areas converges on the entorhinal region and the amygdala. These connections establish the afferent trunk of the limbic loop. In the human brain, the stream of neocortical information thus provides the most important input to the limbic system. Projections from the entorhinal region, amygdala, and hippocampal formation contribute to the efferent trunk of the limbic loop, which heavily influences the prefrontal areas.

the major routes for this transport and incorporate the basal ganglia, select nuclei of the lower brain stem, and the cerebellum into the regulation of cortical output.

The limbic system participates in data transfer and is involved at a critical point where information is transferred from the high order sensory association areas to the prefrontal cortex. One contingent of information leaves the mainstream to converge on the allocortex and amygdala (Fig. 8–2). The transentorhinal region, which abuts the lateral border of the entorhinal cortex, and the lateral nucleus of the amygdala serve as major gates of access for this highly processed neocortical information, which then is distributed to a variety of limbic structures (Fig. 8–3).

The neocortex thus is the chief source of input to the human limbic system. It should be noted that those components of the limbic loop that process neocortical data are a late development both phylogenetically and ontogenetically. In the wake of evolution from macrosmatic mammals to microsmatic higher primates and humans, there occurred not only a remarkable expansion of the neocortex but also a thoroughgoing internal reorganization of limbic loop centers (Fig. 8–4). The major vestige of this change is a massive expansion of components that receive input from and generate output to the neocortex. This increase occurs at the expense of components involved in the processing of olfactory data. The highest directive entities of the limbic loop consist of the entorhinal region, amygdala, and hippocampus. Projections from all three contribute to the efferent trunk of the limbic loop, which, in the human brain, exerts considerable influence on the prefrontal cortex (Fig. 8–3).

In addition, the amygdala receives abundant viscerosensory information and issues projections to major visceromotor nuclei and to nuclei that control endocrine functions. Furthermore, it controls all of the nonthalamic nuclei that generate diffuse and nonspecific projections to the cerebral cortex and other components of the central nervous system (Figs. 8–3, 8–5). These include the cholinergic magnocellular nuclei of the basal forebrain, the GABAergic and histaminergic tuberomammillary nucleus of the hypothalamus, the dopaminergic nuclei of the ventral tegmentum, the noradrenergic locus coeruleus, and the serotonergic anterior raphe nuclei. All of these nuclei exert in-

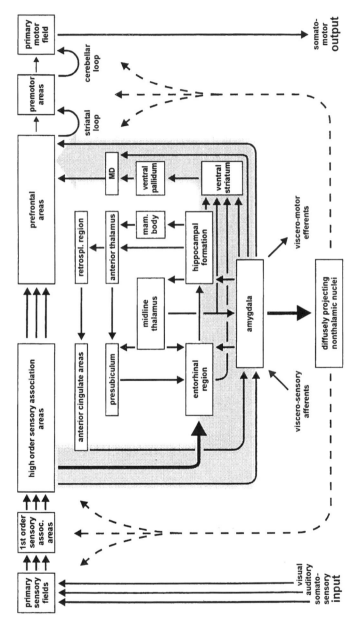

Figure 8–3. The limbic loop is shown in greater detail. The large shaded arrow emphasizes the strategic position of the limbic loop between the neocortical high order sensory association areas and the prefrontal areas. The hippocampal formation, entorhinal region, and amygdala are densely interconnected. Taken together, the three represent the highest directive level of the limbic system. Key: mam.body, mamillary body; MD, mediodorsal thalamic nucleus; retrospl.region, retrosplenial region.

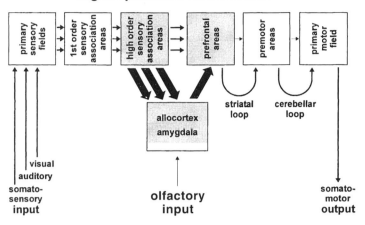

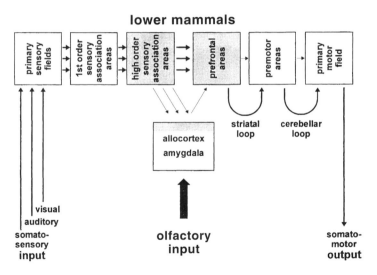

Figure 8–4. Components of the limbic loop that process neocortical data are late developments, both phylogenetically and ontogenetically. In the course of evolution from macrosmatic lower mammals to microsmatic higher primates and humans, a massive expansion of those limbic loop components that receive input from and generate output to the neocortex takes place. This increase occurs at the expense of components processing olfactory data.

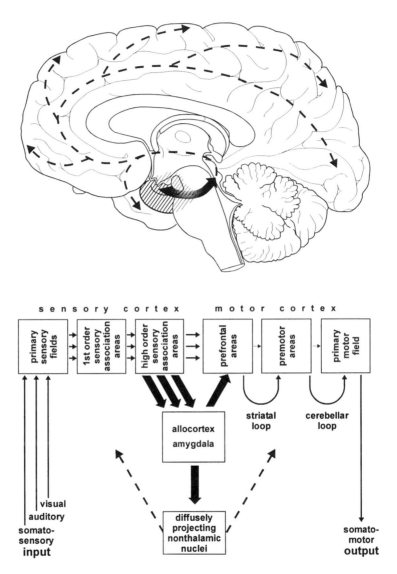

Figure 8–5. The amygdala controls all of the nonthalamic nuclei that generate diffuse and nonspecific projections to the cerebral cortex and other components of the brain and spinal cord. These nuclei include the cholinergic magnocellular nuclei of the basal forebrain, the GABAergic and histaminergic tuberomammillary nucleus of the hypothalamus, the dopaminergic nuclei of the ventral tegmentum, the noradrenergic locus coeruleus, and the serotonergic anterior raphe nuclei. All of these nuclei exert a global influence on the level of activity in their target regions (indicated by broken lines).

fluence on the level of activity in their target regions (Saper, 1987; Nieuwenhuys, 1996).

Myelination and Pigmentation of the Cerebral Cortex and Related Nuclei

A diagram illustrates the fundamental principles that govern myelination and pigmentation within the human central nervous system (Fig. 8–6). Myelination commences prenatally, progresses in an orderly predetermined sequence, and persists well into adulthood. Whereas components of the spinal cord, lower brain stem, and basal ganglia myelinate early, the telencephalic cortex in general and its intracortical lines of Baillarger and Kaes Bechterew in particular undergo a late-onset and prolonged myelination process (Vogt and Vogt, 1919; Flechsig, 1920; Yakovlev and Lecours, 1967).

Initial traces of myelin appear in the primary motor field and in primary sensory fields of the neocortex. The myelination process then continues via the related first order association areas into the high order association areas (Figs. 8–6, 8–7). This results in exceptionally dense myelination (*typus dives*) of the neocortical primary fields in the adult. With increasing distance from the primary fields, a gradational decrease in the average myelin content occurs, and those areals furthest removed, that is, the high order processing areas close to the allocortex, display remarkably poor myelination (*typus pauper*). This areal gradation is an important factor facilitating distinction of architectonic units. The myelin content of neo- and allocortical areas cannot be compared directly because of major structural differences between the two. It is important to point out, however, that allocortical cellular layers are, for the most part, sparsely myelinated and that limbic fiber tracts such as the fornix and the perforant path begin and finish myelination late (Vogt and Vogt, 1919; Flechsig, 1920; Yakovlev and Lecours, 1967; Braak, 1980; Brody et al., 1987; Kinney et al., 1988; van der Knaap et al., 1991; van der Knaap and Valk, 1995).

The average density of cortical intraneuronal pigmentation bears an enigmatic likeness to the negative image of cortical myelination (Braak 1980, 1984). Cortical intraneuronal lipofuscin granules first become apparent in early adulthood, thereafter increasing gradually in number. Richly myelinated cortical areas in the adult human brain, such as the primary motor field as well as cortical layers fortified with a thick plexus of myelinated fibers, are, in general, sparsely pigmented and appear light (*typus clarus*), whereas the extremely sparsely myelinated basal temporal neocortex and the transentorhinal region have a dark appearance (*typus obscurus*) and are among the most richly pigmented territories of the cortex (Braak, 1980) (Fig. 8–7). The projection cells in the superficial entorhinal cellular layer that generate fi-

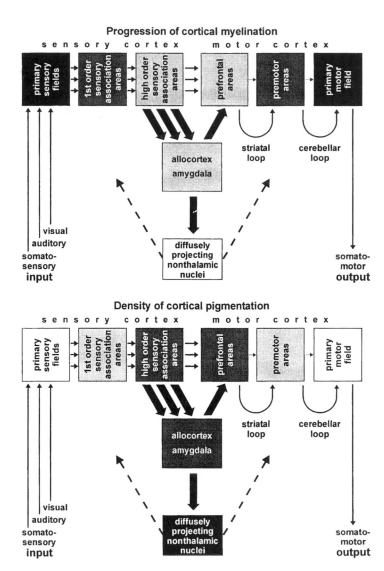

bers of the perforant path are particularly rich in lipofuscin granules. Conspicuous amounts of lipofuscin or neuromelanin also can be observed in the projection cells of all of the above-mentioned non-thalamic nuclei with diffuse nonspecific projections, that is, the magnocellular basal forebrain nuclei, tubero-mamillary nucleus, locus coeruleus, and oral raphe nuclei (Fig. 8–6). Notably, the pigment-laden projection cells of all of these nuclei generate a thin axon that remains unmyelinated or only sparsely myelinated even in adulthood and senescence (Nieuwenhuys, 1996).

AGE-RELATED CHANGES

In the absence of disease-related destruction, the structure of the aging human brain and, in particular, that of the cerebral cortex is maintained at a high level (Creasy and Rapoport, 1985; Peters et al., 1994, 1996, 1997; West et al., 1994; Mrak et al., 1997). Presently available data concerning exclusively age-related changes are controversial (Dickson, 1998a; Hyman and Gómez-Isla, 1998; Finch and Sapolsky, 1999; Victoroff, 1999). The reported changes may represent early (preclinical) stages of AD or other diseases (Davis et al., 1999; Price and Morris, 1999; Green et al., 2000).

←————————

Figure 8–6. *Upper half*: Cortical myelination begins in neocortical primary sensory and primary motor fields and progresses via first order sensory association areas and premotor areas to the related high order association and prefrontal areas. This results in very dense myelination of the neocortical primary sensory and primary motor fields in the human adult. With increasing distance from the primary fields, the average myelin content falls off gradually (indicated by different shading of the boxes). *Lower half*: The average density of cortical intraneuronal pigmentation bears a likeness to the negative image of cortical myelination. In the human adult brain, the neocortical primary fields are sparsely pigmented. With increasing distance from the primary fields, a gradual increase in the average pigment content occurs (indicated by different shading of the boxes: the darker the box, the heavier the pigmentation). Conspicuous amounts of lipofuscin or neuromelanin can be observed in the projection cells of all of the non-thalamic nuclei with diffuse nonspecific projections to the mature neocortex.

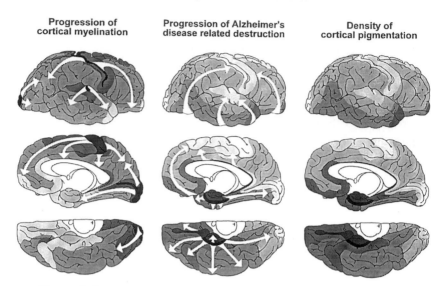

| Progression of cortical myelination | Progression of Alzheimer's disease related destruction | Density of cortical pigmentation |

Figure 8–7. *Left*: The first traces of myelin appear in the primary ne-ocortical fields. The myelination process then progresses via the first order sensory association areas and premotor areas into the related high order association areas (arrows). In the brain of the human adult, the primary fields are remarkably densely myelinated. *Center*: AD-related cortical de-struction begins in the transentorhinal region; from there the pathology extends into adjoining areas, eventually reaching the neocortical primary sensory and motor fields (arrows). *Right*: In the cerebral cortex of the hu-man adult, the average density of intraneuronal pigmentation represents a negative image of the average myelin content. Note that the sequence of destruction resembles the inverse sequence of the cortical myelination pro-cess in early development and is accompanied by a gradual decrease in the average pigment content of cortical nerve cells. Richly myelinated cortical areas are barely pigmented and are the last to develop AD-related changes.

The belief in the inevitability of a substantial age-related loss of nerve cells is widely held. Recent data convincingly show that in humans and in rhesus monkeys, the loss of nerve cells within the normally aging cerebral cortex is either insignificant or much lower than reported earlier (Gómez-Isla et al., 1996, 1997; Hy-man and Gómez-Isla, 1998). As regards subcortical nuclei, only select types of nerve cells display an age-related numerical de-cline, for example, the lipofuscin-laden projection cells of nuclei with diffuse and nonselective projections to the cerebral cortex (Cragg, 1975; Terry et al., 1987; Haug and Eggers, 1991; Peters et al., 1994, 1996, 1997; Wickelgren, 1996a, 1996b; Gazzaley et al., 1997).

The various types of cortical pyramidal cells differ in their susceptibility to age-related alterations. Layer IIIc pyramidal cells in the prefrontal cortex frequently exhibit reductions in the size of their cell bodies, which gradually assume an edged and gnarled appearance (Fig. 8–8b). This transformation usually is not encountered in the sensory association areas. The cytoplasmic density of cortical pyramidal cells increases, and the formerly evenly distributed lipofuscin granules tend to accumulate at the base of the cell body (Fig. 8–8d).

Dendritic processes of specific cortical projection cells occasionally show some irregularities in contour, a loss of spines, and a reduction in number and length (Braak and Braak, 1985; Ruiz-Marcos et al., 1992; Anderson and Rutledge, 1996). In projection cells of the superficial entorhinal cellular layer, a continuous outgrowth of the most distal dendritic segments is observed that lasts well into old age (Buell and Coleman, 1981; Curcio et al., 1982; Coleman and Flood, 1987).

In mature cortical pyramidal cells, the axon hillock and the axon itself normally remain devoid of lipofuscin granules. In old age, however, pigment appears in these two locations in specific types of pyramidal cells (Braak, 1979; Braak et al., 1980). In the initial phase, the axon hillock gradually becomes filled with granules, and shortly thereafter perpendicular rows of lipofuscin granules appear in the proximal axon (Fig. 8–8e). Further accumulation of the pigment eventually leads to the formation of spindle-shaped meganeurites comparable in size and shape to those developing in storage diseases (Fig. 8–8f). The neocortical layer IIIab pyramidal cells are particularly susceptible to such alterations. These easily recognizable changes probably are specific to the human brain since they have yet to be reported in nonhuman mammalian species.

While some areas and layers, for instance the molecular layer of both the subiculum and presubiculum, show prolonged myelination that continues into old age, others reveal a decrease in average myelin content (Kemper, 1984; Meier-Ruge et al., 1992; Raz et al., 1997; Salat et al., 1999). The specific processes underlying the age-associated alterations and the disappearance

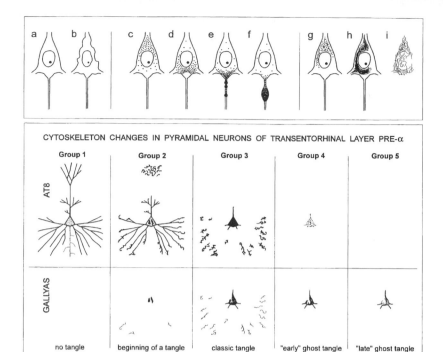

Figure 8–8. *Upper row:* (a) Schematic drawing of a cortical pyramidal cell; (b) in senium, layer IIIc pyramidal cells in the prefrontal cortex exhibit a reduction in the size of their cell bodies; (c) loose distribution of lipofuscin granules in mature layer IIIab pyramidal cells; (d) with age, pigment granules tend to accumulate in basal portions of the cytoplasm; the axon hillock and the axon itself remain devoid of lipofuscin granules; (e) in old age, pigment granules appear in the axon hillock and the proximal axon; (f) gradual accumulation of the pigment leads to the formation of spindle-shaped meganeurites; (g) initial traces of NFT material are seen close to intraneuronal lipofuscin granules; (h) the mature NFT fills the perikaryon and occasionally extends into the proximal dendrites but never into the axon; (i) extraneuronal "ghost" tangle. *Lower portion:* Progression of AD-related alterations of the neuronal cytoskeleton in susceptible cortical pyramidal cells. Sequential changes in the immunoreaction for hyperphosphorylated tau protein (AT8) are displayed for comparison with a corresponding pattern seen in silver-stained sections for demonstration of solid neurofibrillary changes (Gallyas). At first, a soluble hyperphosphorylated tau protein fills the perikaryon and all of the neuronal processes (group 1). In a further step, cross-linkage of the abnormal material takes place and argyrophilic precipitates begin to appear (group 2). The distal dendritic segments become contorted and probably detached from the proximal stem (group 3). Slender NTs develop within the dendrites and an NFT appears in the soma (groups 3 and 4). After deterioration of the parent cell, a "ghost" or "tombstone" tangle remains (group 5). [With permission from E. Braak et al. (1994).]

of cortical myelin are unknown (Dickson et al., 1990, 1991; Peters et al., 1996; Dickson, 1998a). Presumably, the myelin sheaths of thin and inconspicuous axons that finish myelination late and are sparsely myelinated are subject to the most change.

In senium, there appears to be a shift in the balance between neuronal and glial cell populations, with a mild increase in the number of astrocytes (Dickson, 1998a), a feature that is pronounced in the murine brain (O'Callaghan and Miller, 1991; Finch and Day, 1994; Rozovsky et al., 1998). In the human brain, increasing numbers of incidental age-related inclusion bodies known as *corpora amylacea* develop within astrocytic processes close to blood-brain barrier or the cerebrospinal fluid-brain interfaces and in the olfactory bulb (Dickson, 1998a; Kovács et al., 1999). Neuroglial cells in the nonhuman primate brain accumulate inclusions within the cell body that make it easy to distinguish cortical brain tissue of young monkeys from that of old ones by using a light microscope (Peters et al., 1996).

Some components of the human brain are particularly susceptible to the development of disease-related alterations. These do not necessarily and consistently accompany senescence and, as such, must be distinguished carefully from age-affiliated changes. Very frequently, pathological alterations occur that result in the aggregation of "misfolded" proteins at either extracellular, intraneuronal, or intraglial locations (Golbe, 1999; Duda et al., 2000; Lee et al., 2000; Trojanowski and Lee, 2000; Chung et al., 2001). Extracellular deposits appear in the form of β-amyloid proteins and accompanying substances, whereas intraneuronal aggregations include the formation of neurofibrillary tangles, neuropil threads, Lewy bodies, Lewy neurites, Pick bodies, argyrophilic grains, neuronal cytoplasmic inclusions, Hirano bodies, and other insoluble pathological entities (Delacourte et al., 1998; Dickson, 1998a, 1998b; Goedert et al., 1998; Tolnay et al., 1998; Buée and Delacourte, 1999; Goedert, 1999, 2001; Galvin et al., 2001). Comparable changes of the cytoskeleton (e.g., coiled bodies, glial cytoplasmic inclusions) also can be observed in astrocytes and oligodendroglial cells (Braak and Braak, 1989; Yamada and McGeer, 1990; Chin and Goldman, 1996; Feany and Dickson, 1996; Ikeda et al., 1998; Tu et al., 1998; Botez et al., 1999; Dickson et al., 1999). None of these disease-related degenerative changes is part and parcel of the "normal" or successful aging process.

AGE- AND GENDER-RELATED CHANGES

Screening of aged nonselected autopsy brains often reveals the presence of a peculiar type of tau protein–immunopositive cytoskeletal pathology that occurs within the cell bodies and neurites of a class of small, but abundant, nerve cells belonging to the mediobasal hypothalamic region of the human hypothalamo-hypophyseal neurosecretory system (Schultz et al., 1997, 1999). Additional prominent compounds of this pathological profile, which is unique to the aged human mediobasal hypothalamus, are dystrophic cellular processes and perivascular immunoreactive fibers that resemble terminal branches of axons. What is more, a striking correlation exists between the occurrence of these non-AD-related lesions and gender. Whereas women and men under the age of 60 fail to develop the pathology altogether, more than 80% of the men above 75 years of age display the abnormal material; in addition, the most severe forms of the lesions occur exclusively in older men. By comparison, the number of aged women who exhibit the lesions is very small, and the pathology in these cases is milder than that in their male counterparts (Schultz et al., 1997, 1999)

At present, only the human species is known to show this conspicuous as well as enigmatic age- and gender-related predilection for developing tau-associated pathology within the neuroendocrine hypothalamus. Equally remarkable is the fact that the adjacent hypothalamic areas remain virtually uninvolved. The nosological process presumably evolves independently of the process (or processes) underlying AD or the other known tauopathies that often co-occur at an advanced age with the hypothalamic pathology. As such, there are cases of elderly men whose brains are all but devoid of AD-related lesions but contain the tau-protein-immunoreactive material and, *mutatis mutandis*, there are cases of elderly women whose brains exhibit full-blown AD without a trace of the hypothalamic lesions. The mediobasal hypothalamus regulates anterior pituitary functions, and lesions within its infundibular nucleus can be expected to result in gonadal dysfunction (*climacterium virile*).

ALZHEIMER'S DISEASE–RELATED PATHOLOGY

The Degenerative Process

A major criterion, and one that is essential for the neuropathological diagnosis of AD, is assessment of particular cytoskeletal alterations that appear as neurofibrillary tangles (NFTs) in neuronal cell bodies and as neuropil threads (NTs) in dendritic processes. Only a small minority of the many neuronal types that compose the human central nervous system are susceptible to developing these alterations. Attendant changes, which usually develop later in the course of the disease, include β-amyloid protein deposits and neuritic plaques (Beyreuther and Masters, 1991; Braak and Braak, 1991, 1994; Hyman and Gómez-Isla, 1994; Selkoe et al., 1994; Duyckaerts and Hauw, 1997; Esiri et al., 1997; Wegiel and Wisniewski, 1999; Thal et al., 2000). Neurofibrillary tangles/neuropil threads, on the one hand, and β-amyloid precipitations as well as neuritic plaques, on the other, arise independently of each other, and their distribution patterns scarcely overlap (Braak and Braak, 1997, 1999; Spillantini and Goedert, 1998; Price and Morris, 1999).

A decisive turning point in the pathological process is hyperphosphorylation of the tau protein (Grundke-Iqbal et al., 1979, 1986; Goedert et al., 1992, 1997; Goedert, 1993; Köpke et al., 1993; Iqbal et al., 1994, 1998; Duyckaerts et al., 1995; Trojanowski et al., 1995; Alonso et al., 1996; Spillantini and Goedert, 1998; Schneider et al., 1999; Tolnay and Probst, 1999; Buée et al., 2000; Friedhoff et al., 2000). In healthy individuals of all ages, the tau protein stabilizes microtubules. In turn, these components of the neuronal cytoskeleton play an important role in the transport of substances between cellular compartments. With the abnormal phosphorylation of the tau protein, the microtubule assembly becomes disrupted (Grundke-Iqbal et al., 1986; Bramblett et al., 1993; Arendt et al., 1998) and a hydrophilic, non-argyrophilic material arises that fills the perikaryon and all of the neuronal processes (Braak et al., 1994). Initially, the affected cells hardly deviate from their normal shape (Fig. 8–8). Cross-linkage of the abnormal material takes place in a further step, and insoluble argyrophilic precipitates begin to appear (Cras et al., 1995; Smith et al., 1996). At this point, the distal dendritic segments of involved neurons become contorted and dilated; they develop short appendages and likely become detached from the proximal stem (Fig. 8–8). Slender NTs develop within the altered dendrites, and shortly thereafter an NFT appears in the soma (Bancher et al., 1989; Braak et al., 1994; Schwab and McGeer, 1998).

Since the newly formed insoluble and argyrophilic fibrils cannot be degraded by the parent cell, they accumulate and eventually dominate large portions of the neuronal cytoplasm (Fig. 8–8h). The first traces of the abnormal material are closely associated with lipofuscin or neuromelanin granules of the afflicted neurons (Fig. 8–8g). It is possible that the pigment serves as the initiation site for oxidative cross-linking reactions. Other neuronal inclusions such as Lewy bodies or Hirano bodies have no close association with the initial NFTs.

In the cerebral cortex, all NFT-bearing nerve cells belong to the class of pyramidal neurons. Specific types of pyramidal neurons are particularly prone to NFT formation, whereas others are not. Cells that furnish long ipsilateral corticocortical connections are remarkably susceptible to the development of NFTs, whereas inhibitory local circuit neurons generating a short axon are resistant (Lewis et al., 1987; Hof and Morrison, 1991; Hof et al., 1991, 1993; Braak and Braak, 1994, 1999; Morrison and Hof, 1997). In the subcortical nuclei as well, most of the vulnerable cells stand out because of their lengthy axons (German et al., 1987).

Pyramidal cells are sturdy constituents of the cortex and are capable of surviving for decades, despite marked cytoskeletal alterations and changes in neuronal processes (Braak and Braak, 1985; Coleman and Flood, 1987; Bobinksi et al., 1998). The mere preservation of neurons, however, does not mean that their functional capabilities remain intact. Entangled nerve cells probably forfeit much of their functional integrity long before cell death occurs. Subsequent to the final deterioration of the parent cell, the NFT material remains visible in the tissue for years as an extraneuronal "ghost" or "tombstone" tangle, thereby marking the site at which the neuron perished (Siedlak et al., 1991; Braak et al., 1994) (Fig. 8–8i).

The Gradual Evolution of Neurofibrillary Tangles and Neuropil Threads

The destructive process commences in predisposed cortical induction sites, thereafter undermining other portions of the cortex and specific sets of subcortical nuclei in a predictable manner (Kemper, 1978, 1984; Hyman et al., 1984, 1986, 1990; German et al., 1987; van Hoesen and Hyman, 1990; Arnold et al., 1991; Braak and Braak, 1991, 1992, 1994; Price et al., 1991; van Hoesen et al., 1991; Hyman and Gomez-Isla, 1994; Duyckaerts et al., 1997). Assessment of the locations of damaged neurons and of the severity of the pathology provides a conceptual basis for distinguishing the evolutionary stages of the neurofibrillary alterations (Braak and Braak, 1991, 1994, 1997, 1999; Nagy et al., 1995, 1997, 1998; Ohm et al., 1995; Samuel et al., 1996; Hansen and Samuel, 1997; Hyman and Trojanowski, 1997; Ohm, 1997), although such a staging procedure is an artificial construct insofar as the disease-related changes evolve and advance along a continuum rather than in definitive steps (Gertz et al., 1998; Gold et al., 2000; Green et al., 2000).

The transentorhinal region, found in the depths of the rhinal sulcus, is the first cortical region in which the alterations are evident. In stage I only a few entangled neurons are encountered, whereas an accentuated transentorhinal affection plus modest involvement of the entorhinal region proper and the first Ammon's horn sector are seen in stage II (Fig. 8–9). The destruction developing in stages I and II slightly hampers the transmission of neocortical information—via the entorhinal region—to the hippocampal formation (Figs. 8–10, 8–11). Most probably because of interindividual differences with respect to brain neuronal reserves, the severity of the pathological changes may or may not remain below the threshold required for the manifestation of initial symptoms. Although the transentorhinal stages I and II originally were proposed as representing the "silent" phase of AD (Braak and Braak, 1991; Arriagada et al., 1992; Braak et al., 1993; Linn et al., 1995; Nagy et al., 1995; Grober et al., 1999), more recent studies that provide evidence to the contrary underscore the ongoing need to realign the neuropathological staging system on this point with current findings based on the diagnostic or test criteria applied and the cohorts involved (Gold et al., 2000; Jellinger, 2000; Riley et al., 2002).

The characteristic feature of stage III is severe destruction of the transentorhinal and entorhinal regions reflected by the appearance of numerous "ghost" tangles in the affected layers (Gómez-Isla et al., 1996). Less dramatic changes occur in the hippocampus, amygdala, and nonthalamic nuclei with diffuse

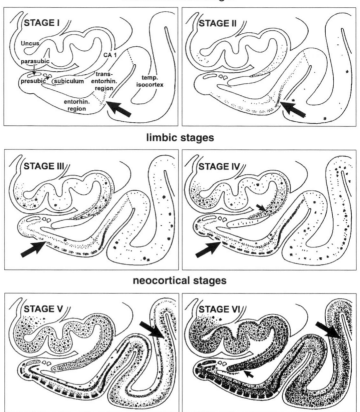

transentorhinal stages

STAGE I — Uncus, parasubic, presubic, (subiculum), trans-entorhin. region, CA 1, temp. isocortex, entorhin. region

STAGE II

limbic stages

STAGE III

STAGE IV

neocortical stages

STAGE V

STAGE VI

Figure 8–9. Summary diagram of the neurofibrillary changes seen—at the level of the uncus—in the hippocampal formation, entorhinal region, transentorhinal region, and adjoining temporal neocortex. Note the development of the lesions from stage I to stage VI (the arrows designate the key features). The pathological alterations start in the transentorhinal region (stage I), then extend into the superficial cellular layer of the entorhinal region (stage II). The limbic stages III and IV show predominant involvement of the entorhinal territory. Destruction of neocortical high-order sensory association and prefrontal areas is the key feature of stage V. The severity of the lesions decreases proceeding from these areas via the first order sensory association and premotor areas into the primary fields of the neocortex. At stage VI, even the sensory primary fields are severely involved. In addition, many granule cells of the fascia dentata develop tangles, and the subiculum displays a remarkably high density of neuropil threads. Key: CA1, first sector of the Ammon's horn; entorhin., entorhinal; parasub., parasubiculum; presubic., presubiculum; temp., temporal; transentorhin., transentorhinal. [With permission from H. Braak and E. Braak (1991).]

and nonspecific projections to the mature neocortex . The latter
remains virtually free of NFTs and NTs (Fig. 8–9). In stage IV,
the neurofibrillary pathology makes inroads into the adjoining
high order association areas of the temporal and insular proneo-
cortices and neocortices (Figs. 8–10, 8–11). A considerable number of persons with stage III or stage IV pathology exhibit amnestic mild cognitive impairment (MCI) (Flicker et al., 1991;
Reisberg and Franssen, 1999; Petersen et al., 1999, 2001; Petersen, 2000)—also referred to as "mild cognitive impairment with
impaired (or delayed) memory" (Riley et al., 2002)—so as to
emphasize the role of incipient memory loss, whereas other cognitive and functional skills, including learning, language, problem solving, judgment or executive functions, concentration, and
the activities of daily living are largely intact despite the presence
of medial temporal lobe neurofibrillary lesions. In other individuals, the appearance of clinical symptoms still may be obscured
by the above-mentioned individual neuronal reserve capacities.
Brain lesions corresponding to stages III or IV have been regarded as representing the morphological counterpart of incipient AD (Jellinger et al., 1991; Bancher et al., 1993, 1996; Braak
et al., 1993; Duyckaerts et al., 1994; Grober et al., 1999).

The meaning of MCI varies, depending on the diagnostic
and other criteria employed to define the term: For some authors, it designates a transitional period between normal, intact
aging and probable or incipient AD (Petersen et al., 1999, 2001;
Petersen, 2000; Riley et al., 2002); for others, it is synonymous
with "very mild" AD, based on the Clinical Dementia Rating
(CDR) scale combined with an alternative neuropathological diagnostic methodology (Morris et al., 2001). Finally, in two recent
studies involving nonagenarians and centenarians, MCI has been
associated, in part, alternately with stages I–II (Gold et al., 2000)
and III (Jellinger, 2000), while stage IV represents in both the
threshold to an overt form of dementia.

The hallmark of AD in stage V is extensive devastation of
the neocortex: The lesions advance superolaterally from the inferior temporal areas, and large numbers of NFTs gradually appear within the high order association areas of the neocortex
(Figs. 8–7, 8–9), where severe disruption of interconnections
between these areas is reflected by widespread synapse loss (Masliah et al., 1993). Only the primary motor field, the primary sen-

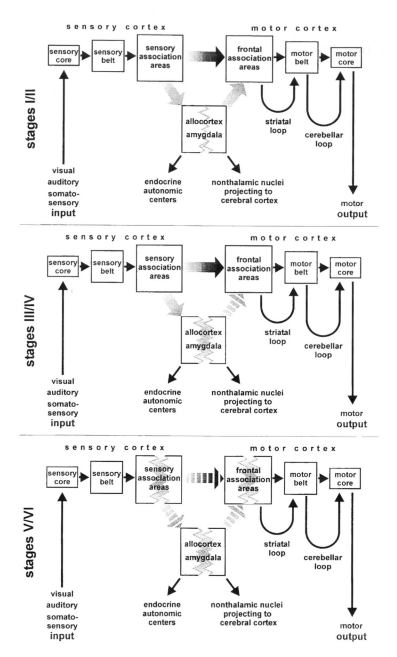

Figure 8–10.

sory fields, and their first order association areas remain un-involved or exhibit minimal destruction. In stage VI, the pathological process even penetrates the primary fields (Figs. 8–10, 8–11). With the degeneration and increasing atrophy of the neocortex in stages V and VI, patients often present with severe dementia (Grober et al., 1999; Gold et al., 2000; Jellinger, 2000; Riley et al., 2002), and major perturbations of autonomic functions reflect the far-reaching destruction of limbic loop centers (Reisberg and Franssen, 1999).

Since 1991, a growing consensus has begun to emerge in the literature, which indicates that the characteristic neuroanatomical substrate of AD, namely, the neurofibrillary pathology, may correlate to a greater degree than β-amyloid deposition with available data pertaining to cognitive deficits and decline, ranging from MCI to varying degrees of dementia in AD (Bancher et al., 1996; Hyman, 1998; Grober et al., 1999; Neuropathology group, 2001; Kay and Roth, 2002; Riley et al., 2002). This trend is not unimportant considering the far-reaching practical implications of potential causal therapeutic strategies designed to inhibit the abnormal conformation of the protein tau prior to the development of the very first β-amyloid plaques in the brain.

Relation of Myelination and Pigmentation to Evolution of AD-Related Lesions

The reasons for the remarkable consistency of the pattern of NFT/NT-related lesions remain enigmatic. Nonetheless, it is likely that the vulnerable types of nerve cells share a number of common properties (Braak et al., 2000). A key to deciphering

←——————————

Figures 8–10 and 8–11. Components of the limbic loop play a significant role in the maintenance of memory functions. Precisely these areas are susceptible to initial pathological changes. Transfer of data from neocortical high order sensory association areas through the limbic loop to the prefrontal areas is impaired early in the course of AD. Further advance of the disorder leads to severe destruction of the neocortical high order sensory association and prefrontal areas. Transfer of data from neocortical high order sensory association areas through long corticocortical pathways to the prefrontal areas is impaired late in the course of AD. Key: mam. body, mamillary body; MD, mediodorsal thalamic nucleus; retrosplen. cortex, retrosplenial cortex. (See Figure 8–11 on next page.)

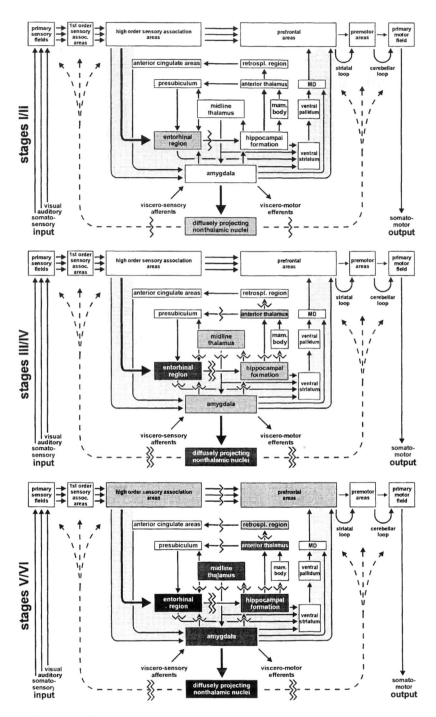

Figure 8–11.

the selective vulnerability and the consistency in the spread of the pathological changes may reside in the striking observation that the AD-related sequence of destruction represents the inverse of the cortical myelination process (Fig. 8–7): Cortical areas and layers that begin myelination late develop NFTs and NTs sooner in the course of AD, and at higher densities, than those that commence myelination early (McGeer et al., 1990; Braak and Braak, 1996). It should be noted in this context that regressive alterations in the brain often recapitulate the process of maturation and refinement but in reverse order (Rapoport, 1988; Bachevalier and Mishkin, 1992; Reisberg et al., 1992; Ruiz-Marcos et al., 1992; Braak and Braak, 1996). Consequently, even in the end stages of AD, all of the cortical or subcortical neurons that develop a long and voluminous axon enclosed in a thick myelin sheath are protected against the development of NFTs and NTs.

Subcortical nuclei particularly prone to develop NFTs and NTs include components of the magnocellular basal forebrain nuclei, the tuberomammillary nucleus, locus coeruleus, and oral raphe nuclei (German et al., 1987; Rüb et al., 2000; Sassin et al., 2000). The projection cells of all of these nuclei are not only heavily pigmented but generate a remarkably thin or unmyelinated axon (Fig. 8–6). Many issues still need to be resolved should the class of projection cells equipped with a long, sparsely myelinated or unmyelinated axon truly include the majority of the nerve cells ultimately involved in AD.

Implications of Staging Data from Nonselected Autopsy Brains for Aging and Alzheimer's Disease–Associated Changes

The relationships among age and NFT/NT-associated alterations can be studied by staging large numbers of nonselected brains at autopsy (Fig. 8–12). In a small number of cases, the initial neurofibrillary changes develop in surprisingly young individuals, that is, in young and otherwise healthy, normal brains. Thus, advanced age in itself is not a prerequisite for their occurrence. Accordingly, the pathological process underlying AD is by no means an age-dependent one. Rather, it is typical of this disorder that several decades elapse between the onset of the lesions and phases of the illness in which the damage is extensive and severe

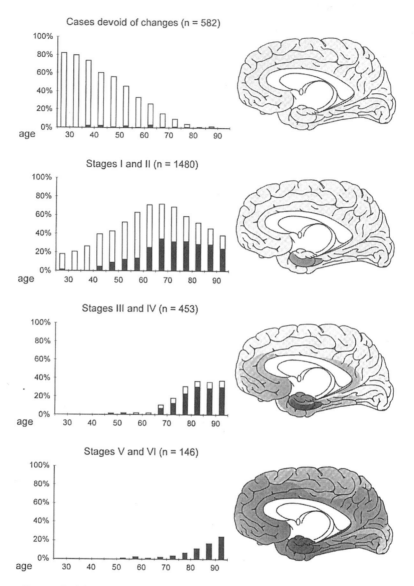

Figure 8–12. Development of AD-related neurofibrillary changes in a total number of 2661 nonselected autopsy cases. The first line displays the frequency of cases devoid of alterations in relation to the total number of cases in the various age categories. The brains of some elderly individuals are free from neurofibrillary pathology. The second, third, and fourth lines are similarly designed and show the evolution of the NFT/NT-related stages. Some individuals develop lesions corresponding to stage I or II early in life. Old age is not a prerequisite for the evolution of the alterations. Note that early stages occur preferably in younger age categories, whereas more advanced stages gradually appear with increasing age. [With permission from H. Braak and E. Braak (1997).]

176

enough for symptoms to become apparent (Ohm et al., 1995; Braak and Braak, 1997; Duyckaerts and Hauw, 1997; Ohm, 1997).

The age spectrum from NFT/NT stages I to VI indicates that early stages occur preferentially in younger age categories, whereas later stages become more prevalent with increasing age. In the final analysis, whether or not the destructive degenerative process underlying AD presents clinically depends largely on whether the longevity and disposition (including perhaps the myelination status) of a given individual allow its expression.

A continuum of the pathological alterations exists, commencing with the first NFT and culminating in the density of lesions seen in fully developed AD. No single feature permits definition of a specific form of the intraneuronal changes related exclusively to age (Dickson et al., 1991; Braak and Braak, 1997). The extremely lengthy time period during which the lesions develop and the fact that they affect a very large proportion of the aging population should neither distract us from their insidious nature nor mislead us to regard them as normal. The same goes for the initial cells of a prostate cancer, which are clinically silent but must be viewed unreservedly as part of a larger pathological event, although such changes are highly prevalent among older men. In other words, an alteration in tissue components can be an extremely commonplace phenomenon, yet still not merit the classification "normal."

NFTs often co-occur with "ghost" tangles. Were periods of remission or spontaneous recovery to occur in AD, two features could be anticipated to characterize the brain tissue of such patients at autopsy: First, the pathological process would persist in all of the involved neurons until the neurons died, thereby resulting in a massive array of "ghost" tangles. Second, still uninvolved nerve cells would have failed to commence generating NFTs prior to death, with the result that only "ghost" tangles would be seen postmortem, thereby indicating that the pathological process had been active for a certain period of time but then ceased. Inasmuch as this scenario has yet to be observed, it can be concluded that the disease process, once initiated, continues right up to the time of death. In spite of the fact that the total nerve cell loss is considerable in clinically overt cases of AD, the AD-related pathology is selective and, accordingly, numerous centers and pathways remain uninvolved even in the final stages of the illness.

Acknowledgments

This work was supported by the Deutsche Forschungsgemeinschaft and the Bundesministerium für Bildung, Wissenschaft, Forschung und Technologie, the Alzheimer Research Center Frankfurt (Alzheimer Forschungs-Zentrum Frankfurt), and Degussa, Hanau. The skillful assistance of Ms. Inge Szász (graphics) is gratefully acknowledged.

References

Alonso, A.C., I. Grundke-Iqbal, and K. Iqbal. (1996). Alzheimer's disease hyperphosphorylated tau sequesters normal tau into tangles of filaments and disassembles microtubules. *Nat Med* 2:783–787.

Anderson, B., and V. Rutledge. (1996). Age and hemisphere effects on dendritic structure. *Brain* 119:1983–1990.

Arendt, T., M. Holzer, R. Fruth, M.K. Brückner, and U. Gärtner. (1998). Phosphorylation of tau, Aβ-formation, and apoptosis after in vivo inhibition of PP-1 and PP-2A. *Neurobiol Aging* 19:3–13.

Arnold, S.E., B.T. Hyman, J. Flory, A.R. Damasio, and G.W. van Hoesen. (1991). The topographical and neuroanatomical distribution of neurofibrillary tangles and neuritic plaques in the cerebral cortex of patients with Alzheimer's disease. *Cerebral Cortex* 1:103–116.

Arriagada, P.V., H.H. Growdon, E.T. Hedley-Whyte, and B.T. Hyman. (1992). Neurofibrillary tangles but not senile plaques parallel duration and severity of Alzheimer disease. *Neurology* 42:631–639.

Bachevalier, J., and M. Mishkin. (1992). Ontogenetic development and decline of memory functions in nonhuman primates. In Neurodevelopment, Aging and Cognition, edited by I. Kostovic, S. Knezevic, H.M. Wisniewski, and G.J. Spillich (pp. 37–59). Boston: Birkhäuser.

Bancher, C., H. Braak, P. Fischer, and K.A. Jellinger. (1993). Neuropathological staging of Alzheimer lesions and intellectual status in Alzheimer's and Parkinson's disease. *Neurosci Lett* 162:179–182.

Bancher, C., C. Brunner, H. Lassmann, H. Budka, K. Jellinger, G. Wiche, F. Seitelberger, I. Grundke-Iqbal, and H.M. Wisniewski. (1989). Accumulation of abnormally phosphorylated tau precedes the formation of neurofibrillary tangles in Alzheimer's disease. *Brain Res* 477:90–99.

Bancher, C., K. Jellinger, H. Lassmann, and P. Fischer. (1996). Correlations between mental state and quantitative neuropathology in the Vienna longitudinal study on dementia. *Eur Arch Psychiatry Clin Neurosci* 246:137–146.

Beyreuther, K., and C.L. Masters. (1991). Amyloid precursor protein (APP) and βA4 amyloid in the etiology of Alzheimer's disease: precursor product relationships in the derangement of neuronal function. *Brain Path* 1:241–252.

Bobinski, M., J. Wegiel, M. Tarnawski, M.J. de Leon, B. Reisberg, D.C. Miller, and H.M. Wisniewski. (1998). Duration of neurofibrillary changes in the hippocampal pyramidal neurons. *Brain Res* 799:156–158.

Botez, G., A. Probst, S. Ipsen, and M. Tolnay. (1999). Astrocytes expressing hyperphosphorylated tau protein without glial fibrillary tangles in argyrophilic grain disease. *Acta Neuropathol* 98:251–256.

Braak, H. (1979). Spindle-shaped appendages of IIIab-pyramids filled with lipofuscin: a striking pathological change of the senescent human isocortex. *Acta Neuropathol* 46:197–202.

Braak, H. (1980). Architectonics of the Human Telencephalic Cortex. Berlin: Springer.

Braak, H. (1984). Architectonics as seen by lipofuscin stains. In Cerebral Cortex, edited by A. Peters and E.G. Jones (Vol. 1, pp. 59–104). New York: Plenum.

Braak, H., and E. Braak. (1985). Golgi preparations as a tool in neuropathology with particular reference to investigations of the human telencephalic cortex. *Progr Neurobiol* 25:93–139.

Braak, H., and E. Braak. (1989). Cortical and subcortical argyrophilic grains characterize a disease associated with adult onset dementia. *Neuropathol Appl Neurobiol* 15:13–26.

Braak, H., and E. Braak. (1991). Neuropathological stageing of Alzheimer-related changes. *Acta Neuropathol* 82:239–259.

Braak, H., and E. Braak. (1992). The human entorhinal cortex: normal morphology and lamina-specific pathology in various diseases. *Neurosci Res* 15:6–31.

Braak, H., and E. Braak. (1994). Pathology of Alzheimer's disease. In Neurodegenerative Diseases, edited by D.B. Calne (pp. 585–613). Philadelphia: Saunders.

Braak, H., and E. Braak. (1996). Development of Alzheimer-related neurofibrillary changes in the neocortex inversely recapitulates cortical myelogenesis. *Acta Neuropathol* 92:197–201.

Braak, H., and E. Braak. (1997). Frequency of stages of Alzheimer-related lesions in different age categories. *Neurobiol Aging* 18:351–357.

Braak, H., and E. Braak. (1999). Temporal sequence of Alzheimer's disease–related pathology. In Cerebral Cortex, Vol. 14: Neurodegenerative and age-related changes in structure and function of the cerebral cortex, edited by A. Peters and J.H. Morrison (pp. 475–512). New York: Kluwer Academic/Plenum.

Braak, E., H. Braak, and E.M. Mandelkow. (1994). A sequence of cytoskeleton changes related to the formation of neurofibrillary tangles and neuropil threads. *Acta Neuropathol* 87:554–567.

Braak, E., H. Braak, H. Strenge, and U. Muhtaroglu. (1980). Age-related alterations of the proximal axon segment in lamina IIIab-pyramidal cells of the human isocortex. A Golgi and fine structural study. *J Hirnforsch* 21:531–535.

Braak, H., K. Del Tredici, C. Schultz, and E. Braak. (2000). Vulnerability of select neuronal types to Alzheimer's disease. *Ann NY Acad Sci* 924:53–61.

Braak, H., C. Duyckaerts, E. Braak, and F. Piette. (1993). Neuropathological staging of Alzheimer-related changes correlates with psychometrically assessed intellectual status. In Alzheimer's Disease: Advances in Clinical and Basic Research, edited by B. Corian, K. Iqbal, M. Nicolini, B. Winblad, H. Wisniewski, and P.F. Zatta (pp. 131–137). Chichester: Wiley.

Bramblett, G.T., M. Goedert, R. Jakes, S.E. Merrick, J.Q. Trojanowski, and V.M.Y. Lee. (1993). Abnormal tau phosphorylation at Ser396 in Alzheimer's disease recapitulates development and contributes to reduced microtuble binding. *Neuron* 10:1089–1099.

Brion, J.J., G. Tremp, and J.N. Octave. (1999). Transgenic expression of the shortest human tau affects its compartmentalization and its phosphorylation as in the pretangle stage of Alzheimer's disease. *Am J Pathol* 154:255–270.

Brody, B.A., H.C. Kinney, A.S. Kloman, and F.H. Gilles. (1987). Sequence of central nervous system myelination in human infancy. I. An autopsy study of myelination. *J Neuropathol Exp Neurol* 46:283–301.

Buée, L., and A. Delacourte. (1999). Comparative biochemistry of tau in progressive supranuclear palsy, corticobasal degeneration, FTDP-17 and Pick's disease. *Brain Pathol* 9:681–693.

Buée, L., T. Bussiere, V. Buée-Scherrer, A. Delacourte, and P.R. Hof. (2000). Tau protein isoforms, phosphorylation and role in neurodegenerative disorders. *Brain Res Rev* 33:95–130.

Buell, S.J., and P.D. Coleman. (1981). Quantitative evidence for selective dendritic growth in normal aging but not in senile dementia. *Brain Res* 214:23–41.

Chin, S.S.M., and J.E. Goldman. (1996). Glial inclusions in CNS degenerative diseases. *J Neuropathol Exp Neurol* 55:499–508.

Chung, K.K.K., V.L. Dawson, and T.M. Dawson. (2001). The role of the ubiquitin-proteasomal pathway in Parkinson's disease and other neurodegenerative disorders. *Trends Neurosci* 24:7–14.

Coleman, P.D., and D.G. Flood. (1987). Neuron numbers and dendritic extent in normal aging and Alzheimer's disease. *Neurobiol Aging* 8:521–545.

Cragg, B.G. (1975). The density of synapses and neurons in normal, mentally defective, and aging human brains. *Brain* 98:81–90.

Cras, P., M.A. Smith, P.L. Richey, S.L. Siedlak, P. Mulvihill, and G. Perry. (1995). Extracellular neurofibrillary tangles reflect neuronal loss and provide further evidence of extensive protein cross-linking in Alzheimer's disease. *Acta Neuropathol* 89:291–295.

Creasey, H., and S.L. Rapoport. (1985). The aging human brain. *Ann Neurol* 17:2–10.

Curcio, C.A., S.J. Buell, and P.D. Coleman. (1982). Morphology of the aging central nervous system: Not all downhill. In The Aging Motor System: Advances in Neurogerontology, edited by J.A. Mortimer, F.J. Pirozollo, and G.J. Maletta (Vol. 3). New York: Praeger.

Davis, D.G., F.A. Schmitt, D.R. Wekstein, and W.R. Markesbery. (1999). Alzheimer neuropathologic alteration in aged cognitively normal subjects. *J Neuropathol Exp Neurol* 58:376–388.

Delacourte, A., N. Sergeant, A. Wattez, D. Gauvreau, and Y. Robitaille. (1998). Vulnerable neuronal subsets in Alzheimer's and Pick's disease are distinguished by their tau isoform distribution and phosphorylation. *Ann Neurol* 43:193–204.

Dickson, D.W. (1998a). Aging in the central nervous system. In Neuropathology of Dementing Disorders, edited by W.R. Markesbery (pp. 56–88). London: Arnold.

Dickson, D.W. (1998b). Pick's disease: a modern approach. Brain Pathol 8: 339–454.

Dickson, D.W., H.A. Crystal, L.A. Mattiace, D.M. Masur, A.D. Blau, P. Davies, S.H. Yen, and M.K. Aronson. (1991). Identification of normal and pathological aging in prospectively studied nondemented elderly humans. Neurobiol Aging 13:179–189.

Dickson, D.W., W. Lin, W.K. Liu, and S.H. Yen. (1999). Multiple system atrophy: a sporadic synucleinopathy. Brain Pathol 9:721–732.

Dickson, D.W., A. Wertkin, Y. Kress, H. Ksiezak-Reding, and S.H. Yen. (1990). Ubiquitin immunoreactive structures in normal brains: distribution and developmental aspects. Lab Invest 63:87–99.

Duda, J.E., V.M.Y. Lee, and J.Q. Trojanowski. (2000). Neuropathology and synuclein aggregates: new insights into mechanism of neurodegenerative diseases. J Neurosci Res 61:121–127.

Duyckaerts, C., M. Bennecib, Y. Grignon, T. Uchihara, Y. He, F. Piette, and J.J. Hauw. (1997). Modeling the relation between neurofibrillary tangles and intellectual status. Neurobiol Aging 18:267–273.

Duyckaerts, C., P. Delaère, Y. He, S. Camilleri, H. Braak, F. Piette, and J.J. Hauw. (1995). The relative merits of tau- and amyloid markers in the neuropathology of Alzheimer's disease. In Treating Alzheimer's and Other Dementias, edited by M. Bergener and S.I. Finkel (pp. 81–89). New York: Springer.

Duyckaerts, C., and J.J. Hauw. (1997). Prevalence, incidence and duration of Braak's stages in the general population: can we know? Neurobiol Aging 18:362–369.

Duyckaerts, C., Y. He, D. Seilhean, P. Delaère, F. Piette, H. Braak, and J.J. Hauw. (1994). Diagnosis and staging of Alzheimer's disease in a prospective study involving aged individuals. Neurobiol, Aging (Suppl 1) 15: 140–141.

Esiri, M.M., B.T. Hyman, K. Beyreuther, and C. Masters. (1997). Aging and dementia. In Greenfield's Neuropathology, edited by D.L. Graham and P.I. Lantos (pp. 153–233). London: Arnold.

Feany, M.B., and D.W. Dickson. (1996). Neurodegenerative disorders with extensive tau pathology: a comparative study and review. Ann Neurol 40:139–148.

Feldman, M.L. (1984). Morphology of the neocortical pyramidal neuron. In Cerebral Cortex, edited by A. Peters and E.G. Jones (Vol. 1, pp. 123–200). New York: Plenum.

Finch, C.E., and J.R. Day. (1994). Molecular biology of aging in the nervous system: a synopsis of the levels of mechanisms. In Neurodegenerative Diseases, edited by D.B. Calne (pp. 33–50). Philadelphia: Saunders.

Finch, C.E., and R.M. Sapolsky. (1999). The evolution of Alzheimer disease, the reproductive schedule, and apoE isoforms. Neurobiol Aging 20:407–428.

Flechsig, P. (1920). Anatomie des menschlichen Gehirns und Rückenmarks auf myelogenetischer Grundlage. Leipzig: Thieme.

Flicker, C., S.H. Ferris, and B. Reisberg. (1991). Mild cognitive impairment in the elderly: predictors of dementia. *Neurology* 41:1006–1009.

Friedhoff, P., M. von Bergen, E.M. Mandelkow, and E. Mandelkow. (2000). Structure of tau protein and assembly into paired helical filaments. *Biochim Biophys Acta* 1502:122–132.

Galvin, J.E., V.M.Y. Lee, and J.Q. Trojanowski. (2001). Synucleinopathies. Clinical and pathological implications. *Arch Neurol* 58:186–190.

Gazzaley, A.H., M.M. Thakker, P.R. Hof, and J.H. Morrison. (1997). Preserved number of entorhinal cortex layer II neurons in aged macaque moneys. *Neurobiol Aging* 18:549–553.

German, D.C., C.L. White, and D.R. Sparkman, (1987). Alzheimer's disease: neurofibrillary tangles in nuclei that project to the cerebral cortex. *Neuroscience* 21:305–312.

Gertz, H.J., J.H. Xuereb, F.A. Huppert, C. Brayne, M.A. McGee, E.S. Paykel, C. Harrington, E. Mukaetova-Ladinska, T. Arendt, and C.M. Wischik. (1998). Examination of the validity of the hierarchical model of neuropathological staging in normal aging and Alzheimer's disease. *Acta Neuropathol* 95:154–158.

Goedert, M. (1993). Tau protein and the neurofibrillary pathology of Alzheimer's disease. *Trends Neurosci* 16:460–465.

Goedert, M. (1999). Filamentous nerve cell inclusion in neurodegenerative diseases: tauopathies and alpha-synucleinopathies. *Phil Trans R Soc Lond B Biol Sci* 354:1101–1118.

Goedert, M. (2001). Alpha-synuclein and neurodegenerative disease. *Nat Rev* 2:492–501.

Goedert, M., M.G. Spillantini, N.J. Cairns, and R.A. Crowther. (1992). Tau proteins from Alzheimer paired helical filaments: abnormal phosphorylation of all six isoforms. *Neuron* 8:159–168.

Goedert, M., M.G. Spillantini, and S.W. Davis. (1998). Filamentous nerve cell inclusions in neurodegenerative diseases. *Curr Opin Neurobiol* 8: 619–632.

Goedert, M., J.Q. Trojanowski, and V.M.Y. Lee. (1997). The neurofibrillary pathology of Alzheimer's disease. In The Molecular and Genetic Basis of Neurological Disease, 2nd ed., edited by R.N. Rosenberg (pp. 613–627). Boston: Butterworth-Heinemann.

Golbe, L.I. (1999). Alpha-synuclein and Parkinson's disease. *Movement Disord* 14:6–9.

Gold, G., C. Bouras, E. Kövari, A. Canuto, B. González Glaría, A. Malky, P.R. Hof, J.P. Michel, and P. Giannakopoulos. (2000). Clinical validity of Braak neuropathological staging in the oldest-old. *Acta Neuropathol* 99:579–582.

Götz, J. (2001). Tau and transgenic animal models. *Brain Res Rev* 35:266–286.

Gómez-Isla, T., R. Hollister, H. West, S. Mui, J.J. Growdon, R.C. Petersen, J.E. Parisi, and B.T. Hyman. (1997). Neuronal loss correlates with but exceeds neurofibrillary tangles in Alzheimer's disease. *Ann Neurol* 41: 17–24.

Gómez-Isla, T., J.L. Price, D.W. McKeel, J.C. Morris, J.H. Growdon, and B.T. Hyman. (1996). Profound loss of layer II entorhinal cortex neurons occurs in very mild Alzheimer's disease. *J Neurosci* 16:4491–4500.

Green, M.S., J.A. Kaye, and M.J. Ball. (2000). The Oregon brain aging study: neuropathology accompanying healthy aging in the oldest old. *Neurology* 54:105–113.

Grober, E., D. Dickson, M.J. Sliwinski, H. Buschke, M. Katz, H. Crystal, and R.B. Lipton. (1999). Memory and mental status correlates of modified Braak staging. *Neurobiol Aging* 20:573–579.

Grundke-Iqbal, I., K. Iqbal, Y. Tung, M. Quinlan, H. Wisniewski, and L. Binder. (1986). Abnormal phosphorylation of the microtubule-associated protein τ (tau) in Alzheimer cytoskeletal pathology. *Proc Natl Academy Sci USA* 83:4913–4917.

Grundke-Iqbal, I., A. Johnson, H. Wisniewski, L. Terry, and K. Iqbal. (1979). Evidence that Alzheimer neurofibrillary tangles originate from neurotubules. *Lancet* 1:578–580.

Hansen, L.A., and W. Samuel. (1997). Criteria for Alzheimer's disease and the nosology of dementia with Lewy bodies. *Neurology* 48:126–132.

Haug, H., and R. Eggers. (1991). Morphometry of the human cortex cerebri and corpus striatum during aging. *Neurobiol Aging* 12:336–338.

Hof, P.R., K. Cox, W.G. Young, M.R. Celio, J. Rogers, and J.H. Morrison. (1991). Parvalbumin-immunoreactive neurons in the neocortex are resistant to degeneration in Alzheimer's disease. *J Neuropathol Exp Neurol* 50:451–462.

Hof, P.R., and J.H. Morrison. (1991). Neocortical neuronal subpopulations labeled by a monoclonal antibody to calbindin exhibit differential vulnerability in Alzheimer's disease. *Exp Neurol* 111:293–301.

Hof, P.R., E.A. Nimchinsky, M.R. Celio, C. Bouras, and J.H. Morrison. (1993). Calretinin-immunoreactive neocortical interneurons are unaffected in Alzheimer's disease. *Neurosci Lett* 152:145–149.

Hyman, B.T. (1998). New neuropathological criteria for Alzheimer's disease. *Arch Neurol* 55:1174–1176.

Hyman, B.T., and T. Gómez-Isla. (1994). Alzheimer's disease is a laminar, regional, and neural system specific disease, not a global brain disease. *Neurobiol Aging* 15:353–354.

Hyman, B.T., and T. Gómez-Isla. (1998). Normal aging and Alzheimer's disease. In Handbook of the Aging Brain, edited by E. Wang and D.S. Snyder. San Diego and London: Academic Press.

Hyman, B.T., and J.Q. Trojanowski. (1997). Editorial on consensus recommendations for the postmortem diagnosis of Alzheimer disease from the National Institute on Aging and the Reagan Institute Working Group on diagnostic criteria for the neuropathological assessment of Alzheimer disease. *J Neuropathol Exp Neurol* 56:1095–1097.

Hyman, B.T., G.W. van Hoesen, and A.R. Damasio. (1990). Memory-related systems in Alzheimer's disease: an anatomic study. *Neurology* 40:1721–1730.

Hyman, B.T., G.W. van Hoesen, A.R. Damasio, and C.L. Barnes. (1984). Alzheimer's disease: cell-specific pathology isolates the hippocampal formation. *Science* 225:1168–1170.

Hyman, B.T., G.W. van Hoesen, L.J. Kromer, and A.R. Damasio. (1986). Perforant pathway changes and the memory impairment of Alzheimer's disease. *Ann Neurol* 20:472–481.

Ikeda, K., H. Akiyama, T. Arai, and T. Nishimura. (1998). Gial tau pathology in neurodegenerative diseases: their nature and comparison with neuronal tangles. *Neurobiol Aging* 19:S85–S91.

Iqbal, K., A.C. Alonso, C.X. Gong, S. Khatoon, J.J. Pei, J.Z. Wang, and I. Grundke-Iqbal. (1998). Mechanisms of neurofibrillary degeneration and the formation of neurofibrillary tangles. *J Neurol Transm* (Suppl) 53:169–180.

Iqbal, K., A.C. Alonso, C.X. Gong, S. Khatoon, T.J. Singh, and I. Grundke-Iqbal. (1994). Mechanism of neurofibrillary degeneration in Alzheimer's disease. *Mol Neurobiol* 9:119–123.

Janus, C., and D. Westaway. (2001). Transgenic mouse models of Alzheimer's disease. *Physiol Behav* 73:873–886.

Jellinger, K. (2000). Clinical validity of Braak staging in the oldest old. *Acta Neuropathol* 99:583–584.

Jellinger, K., H. Braak, E. Braak, and P. Fischer. (1991). Alzheimer lesions in the entorhinal region and isocortex in Parkinson's and Alzheimer's diseases. *Ann NY Acad Sci* 640:203–209.

Kay, D.W.K., and M. Roth. (2002). Pathological correlates of dementia. *Lancet* 359:624–625.

Kemper, T.L. (1978). Senile dementia: a focal disease in the temporal lobe. In Senile Dementia: A Biomedical Approach, edited by E. Nandy (pp. 105–113). Amsterdam: Elsevier.

Kemper, T.L. (1984). Neuroanatomical and neuropathological changes in normal aging and in dementia. In Clinical Neurology of Aging, edited by M.L. Albert (pp. 9–52). Oxford: University Press.

Kinney, H.C., B.A. Brody, A.S. Kloman, and F.H. Gilles. (1988). Sequence of central nervous system myelination in human infancy. II. Patterns of myelination in autopsied infants. *J Neuropathol Exp Neurol* 47:217–234.

Köpke, E., Y.C. Tung, S. Shaikh, A.D. Alonso, K. Iqbal, and I. Grundke-Iqbal. (1993). Microtubule-associated protein tau—abnormal phosphorylation of a non-paired helical filament pool in Alzheimer's disease. *J Biol Chem* 268:24374–24384.

Kovács, T., N.J. Cairns, and P.L. Lantos. (1999). β-Amyloid deposition and neurofibrillary tangle formation in the olfactory bulb in ageing and Alzheimer's disease. *Neuropathol Appl Neurobiol* 25:481–491.

Lee, V.M.-Y., J.Q. Trojanowski, L. Buée, and Y. Christen (eds). (2000). Fatal Attractions—Protein Aggregates in Neurodegenerative Diseases (pp. 1–140). Berlin: Springer.

Lewis, D.A., M.J. Campbell, R.D. Terry, and J.H. Morrison. (1987). Laminar and regional distributions of neurofibrillary tangles and neuritic plaques in Alzheimer's disease: a quantitative study of visual and auditory cortices. *J Neurosci* 7:1799–1808.

Linn, R.T., P.A. Wolf, D.L. Bachman, J.E. Knoefel, J.L. Cobb, A.J. Belanger, E.F. Kaplan, and R.B. D'Agostino. (1995). The "preclinical phase" of probable Alzheimer's disease. A 13-year prospective study of the Framingham cohort. *Arch Neurol* 52:485–490.

Mandelkow, E., and E.M. Mandelkow. (1996). Microtubules and microtubule-associated proteins. *Curr Opin Cell Biol* 7:72–81.

Masliah, E., A. Miller, and R.D. Terry. (1993). The synaptic organization of the neocortex in Alzheimer's disease. *Med Hypotheses* 41:334–340.

McGeer, P.L., E.G. McGeer, H. Akiyama, S. Itagaki, R. Harrop, and R. Peppard. (1990). Neuronal degeneration and memory loss in Alzheimer's disease and aging. *Exp Brain Res* (Suppl) 21:411–426.

Meier-Ruge, W., J. Ulrich, M. Brühlmann, and E. Meier. (1992). Age-related white matter atrophy in the human brain. *Ann NY Acad Sci* 673:260–269.

Morris, J.C., M. Storandt, J.P. Miller, D.W. McKeel, J.L. Price, E.H. Rubin, and L. Berg. (2001). Mild cognitive impairment represents early-stage Alzheimer disease. *Arch Neurol* 58:397–405.

Morrison, J.H., and P.R. Hof. (1997). Life and death of neurons in the aging brain. *Science* 278:412–419.

Mrak, R.E., W.S.T. Griffin, and D.L. Graham. (1997). Aging-associated changes in human brain. *J Neuropathol Exp Neurol* 56:1269–1275.

Nagy, Z.S., M. Esiri, K. Jobst, J. Morris, E.F. King, B. McDonald, S. Litchfield, A. Smith, L. Barnetson, and A.D. Smith. (1995). Relative roles of plaques and tangles in the dementia of Alzheimer's disease: correlations using three sets of neuropathological criteria. *Dementia* 6:21–31.

Nagy, Z.S., B. Vatter-Bittner, H. Braak, F. Braak, D. Yilmazer, C. Schultz, and J. Hanke. (1997). Staging of Alzheimer-type pathology: an interrater-intrarater study. *Dementia* 8:248–251.

Nagy, Z.S., D.M. Yilmazer-Hanke, H. Braak, E. Braak, C. Schultz, and J. Hanke. (1998). Assessment of the pathological stages of Alzheimer's disease in thin paraffin sections: a comparative study. *Dementia* 9:140–144.

Neuropathology Group of the Medical Research Council Cognitive Function and Aging Study (MRC CFAS). (2001). Pathological correlates of late-onset dementia in a multicenter, community-based population study in England and Wales. *Lancet* 357:169–175.

Nieuwenhuys, R. (1994). The neocortex: an overview of its evolutionary development, structural organization and synaptology. *Anat Embryol* 190:307–337.

Nieuwenhuys, R. (1996). The greater limbic system, the emotional motor system and the brain. *Progr Brain Res* 107:551–580.

O'Callaghan, J.P., and D.B. Miller. (1991). The concentration of glial fibrillary acidic protein increases with age in the mouse and rat brain. *Neurobiol Aging* 12:171–174.

Ohm, T.G. (1997). Does Alzheimer's disease start early in life? *Mol Psychiatry* 2:21–25.

Ohm, T.G., H. Müller, H. Braak, and J. Bohl. (1995). Close-meshed prevalence rates of different stages as a tool to uncover the rate of Alzheimer's disease–related neurofibrillary changes. *Neuroscience* 64:209–217.

Peters, A., D. Leahu, M.B. Moss, and K. McNally. (1994). The effects of aging on area 46 of the frontal cortex of the aging monkey. *Cerebral Cortex* 6:621–635.

Peters, A., N.J. Nigro, and K.J. McNally. (1997). A further evaluation of the effect of age on striate cortex of the rhesus monkey. *Neurobiol Aging* 18:29–36.

Peters, A., D.L. Rosene, M.B. Moss, T.L. Kemper, C.R. Abraham, J. Tigges, and M.S. Albert. (1996). Neurobiological bases of age-related cognitive decline in the rhesus monkey. *J Neuropathol Exp Neurol* 55:861–874.

Petersen, R.C. (2000). Mild cognitive impairment: transition between aging and Alzheimer's disease. *Neurologia* 15:93–101.

Petersen, R.C., R. Doody, A. Kurz, R.C. Mohs, J.C. Morris, P.V. Rabins, K. Ritchie, M. Rossor, L. Thal, and B. Winblad. (2001). Current concepts in mild cognitive impairment. *Arch Neurol* 58:1985–1992.

Petersen, R.C., G.E. Smith, S.C. Waring, R.J. Ivnik, E.G. Tangalos, and E. Kokmen. (1999). Mild cognitive impairment: clinical characterization and outcome. *Arch Neurol* 56:303–308.

Price, J.L., P.B. Davis, J.C. Morris, and D.L. White. (1991). The distribution of tangles, plaques and related immunohistochemical markers in healthy aging and Alzheimer's disease. *Neurobiol Aging* 12:295–312.

Price, J.L., and J.C. Morris. (1999). Tangles and plaques in nondemented aging and "preclinical" Alzheimer's disease. *Ann Neurol* 45:358–368.

Rapoport, S.I. (1988). Brain evolution and Alzheimer's disease. *Rev Neurol (Paris)* 144:79–90.

Raz, N., F.M. Gunning, D. Head, J.H. Dupuis, J. McQuain, S.D. Briggs, W.J. Loken, A.E. Thorton, and J.D. Acker. (1997). Selective aging of the human cerebral cortex observed in vivo: differential vulnerability of the prefrontal gray matter. *Cerebral Cortex* 7:268–282.

Reisberg, B., and E.H. Franssen. (1999). Clinical stages of Alzheimer's disease. In An Atlas of Alzheimer's Disease. The Encyclopedia of Visual Medicine, edited by M.J. de Leon (pp. 11–20). New York and London: Parthenon.

Reisberg, B., A. Pattschull-Furlan, E. Franssen, S.G. Sclan, A. Kluger, L. Dingcong, and S.H. Ferris. (1992). Dementia of the Alzheimer type recapitulates ontogeny inversely on specific ordinal and temporal parameters. In Neurodevelopment, Aging and Cognition, edited by I. Kostovic, S. Knezevic, H.M. Wisniewski, and G.J. Spillich (pp. 345–369). Boston: Birkhäuser.

Riley, K.P., D.A. Snowdon, and W.R. Markesbery. (2002). Alzheimer's neurofibrillary pathology and the spectrum of cognitive function: findings from the nun study. *Ann Neurol* 51:567–577.

Roszovsky, I., C.E. Finch, and T.E. Morgan. (1998). Age-related activation of microglia and astrocytes: in vitro studies show persistent phenotypes of aging, increased proliferation, and resistance to down-regulation. *Neurobiol Aging* 19:97–103.

Rüb, U., K. Del Tredici, C. Schultz, D.R. Thal, E. Braak, and H. Braak. (2000). The evolution of Alzheimer's disease–related cytoskeletal pathology in the human raphe nuclei. *Neuropathol Appl Neurobiol* 26:553–557.

Ruiz-Marcos, A., F. Sanchez-Toscano, and J.A. Munoz-Cueto. (1992). Aging reverts to juvenile conditions the synaptic connectivity of cerebral cortical pyramidal shafts. *Dev Brain Res* 69:41–49.

Salat, D.H., P.A. Stangl, J.A. Kaye, and J.S. Janowsky. (1999). Sex differences in prefrontal volume with aging and Alzheimer's disease. *Neurobiol Aging* 20:591–596.

Samuel, W., D. Galasko, E. Masliah, and L.A. Hansen. (1996). Neocortical Lewy body counts correlate with dementia in the Lewy body variant of Alzheimer's disease. *J Neuropathol Exp Neurol* 55:44–52.

Saper, C.B. (1987). Diffuse cortical projection systems: anatomical organization and role in cortical function. In Handbook of Physiology. The Nervous System, edited by F. Plum (Vol. 5, pp. 169–210). Bethesda: American Physiological Society.

Sassin, I., C. Schultz, D.R. Thal, U. Rüb, K. Arai, D. Koppers, E. Braak, and H. Braak. (2000). Evolution of Alzheimer's disease–related cytoskeletal changes in the basal nucleus of Meynert. *Acta Neuropathol* 100:259–269.

Schneider, A., J. Biernat, M. von Bergen, E. Mandelkow, and E.M. Mandelkow. (1999). Phosphorylation that detaches tau protein from microtubles (Ser262, Ser214) also protects it against aggregation into Alzheimer paired helical filaments. *Biochemistry* 38:3549–3558.

Schultz, C., F. Dehghani, G.B. Hubbard, G. Struckhoff, D.R. Thal, E. Braak, and H. Braak. (2000a). Filamentous tau pathology in nerve cells, astrocytes and oligodendrocytes of aged baboons. *J Neuropathol Exp Neurol* 59:39–52.

Schultz, C., E. Ghebremedhin, E. Braak, and H. Braak. (1999). Sex-dependent cytoskeletal changes of the human hypothalamus develop independently of Alzheimer's disease. *Exp Neurol* 160:186–193.

Schultz, C., G.B. Hubbard, E. Braak, and H. Braak. (2000b). Age-related accumulation of abnormally phosphorylated tau protein in neurons and glial cells of baboons. *Neurobiol Aging* 21:905–911.

Schultz, C., D. Koppers, E. Braak, and H. Braak. (1997). Neurofibrillary degeneration in hypophysiotropic nuclei of the aging human hypothalamus. In Neuroendocrinology: Retrospect and Perspectives, edited by H.W. Korf and K.H. Usadel (pp. 115–126). Berlin, Heidelberg: Springer.

Schwab, C., and P.L. McGeer. (1998). Tubulin immunopositive structures resembling intracellular neurofibrillary tangles. *Neurobiol Aging* 19:41–45.

Seabrook, G.R., and T.W. Rosahl. (1999). Transgenic animals relevant to Alzheimer's disease. *Neuropharmacology* 38:1–17.

Selkoe, D.J. (1994). Alzheimer's disease: a central role for amyloid. *J Neuropathol Exp Neurol* 53:438–447.

Siedlak, S.L., P. Cras, M. Kawai, P. Richey, and G. Perry. (1991). Basic fibroblast growth factor binding is a marker for extracellular neurofibrillary tangles in Alzheimer's disease. *J. Histochem Cytochem* 39:899–904.

Smith, M.A., S.L. Siedlak, P.L. Richey, R.H. Nagaraj, A. Elhammer, and G. Perry. (1996). Quantitative solubilization and analysis of insoluble paired helical filaments from Alzheimer disease. *Brain Res* 717:99–108.

Spillantini, M.G., and M. Goedert. (1998). Tau protein pathology in neurodegenerative diseases. *Trends Neurosci* 21:428–433.

Terry, R.D., R. DeTeresa, and L.A. Hansen. (1987). Neocortical cell counts in normal human adult aging. *Ann Neurol* 21:530–539.

Thal, D.R., U. Rüb, C. Schultz, I. Sassin, E. Ghebremedhin, K. Del Tredici, E. Braak, and H. Braak. (2000). Sequence of Aβ-protein deposition in the human medial temporal lobe. *J. Neuropathol Exp Neurol* 59: 733–748.

Tolnay, M., C. Mistl, S. Ipsen, and A. Probst. (1998). Argyrophilic grains of Braak: occurrence in dendrites of neurons containing hyperphosphorylated tau protein. *Neuropathol Appl Neurobiol* 24:53–59.

Tolnay, M., and A. Probst. (1999). Tau protein pathology in Alzheimer's disease and related disorders. *Neuropathol Appl Neurobiol* 25:171–187.

Trojanowski, J.Q., and V.M.-Y. Lee. (2000). "Fatal attractions" of proteins: a comprehensive hypothetical mechanism underlying Alzheimer's disease and other neurodegenerative disorders. *Ann NY Acad Sci* 924:62–67.

Trojanowski, J.Q., R.W. Shin, M.L. Schmidt, and V.M.Y. Lee. (1995). Relationship between plaques, tangles, and dystrophic processes in Alzheimer's disease. *Neurobiol Aging* 16:335–340.

Tu, P.H., J.E. Galvin, M. Baba, B. Giasson, T. Tomita, S. Leight, T. Nakajo, T. Iwatsubo, J.Q. Trojanowski, and V.M.Y. Lee. (1998). Glial cytoplasmic inclusions in white matter oligodendrocytes of multiple system atrophy brains contain insoluble α-synuclein. *Ann Neurol* 44:415–422.

van der Knaap, M.S., and J. Valk. (1995). Magnetic Resonance of Myelin, Myelination, and Myelin Disorders, 2nd ed. Berlin: Springer.

van der Knaap, M.S., J. Valk, C.J. Bakker, M. Schooneveld, J.A.J. Faber, J. Willemse, and R.H.J.M. Gooskens. (1991). Myelination as an expression of the functional maturity of the brain. *Dev Med Child Neurol* 33: 849–857.

van Hoesen, G.W., and B.T. Hyman. (1990). Hippocampal formation: anatomy and the patterns of pathology in Alzheimer's disease. *Progr Brain Res* 83:445–457.

van Hoesen, G.W., B.T. Hyman, and A.R. Damasio. (1991). Entorhinal cortex pathology in Alzheimer's disease. *Hippocampus* 1:1–8.

Victoroff, J. (1999). The evolution of aging-related brain change. *Neurobiol Aging* 20:431–438.

Vogt, C., and O. Vogt. (1919). Allgemeinere Ergebnisse unserer Hirnforschung. *J Psychol Neurol* 25:277–462.

Wegiel, J., and H.M. Wisniewski. (1999). β-Amyloidosis in Alzheimer's disease. In An Atlas of Alzheimer's Disease. The Encyclopedia of Visual Medicine Series, edited by M.J. de Leon (pp. 89–107). New York and London: Parthenon.

West, M.J., P.D. Coleman, D.G. Flood, and J.C. Troncosco. (1994). Differences in the pattern of hippocampal neuronal loss in normal aging and Alzheimer's disease. *Lancet* 344:769–772.

Wickelgren, I. (1996a). Is hippocampal cell death a myth? *Science* 271:1229–1230.

Wickelgren, I. (1996b). The aging brain. For the cortex, neuron loss may be less than thought. *Science* 273:48–50.

Yakovlev, P.I., and A.R. Lecours. (1967). The myelogenetic cycles of regional maturation of the brain. In Regional Development of the Brain in Early Life, edited by A. Minkowksi (pp. 3–70). Oxford: Blackwell.

Yamada, T., and P.L. McGeer. (1990). Oligodendroglial microtubular masses: an abnormality observed in some human neurodegenerative diseases. *Neurosci Lett* 120:163–166.

Zilles, K. (1990). Cortex. In The Human Nervous System, edited by G. Paxinos (pp. 757–802). New York: Academic Press.

CHAPTER **9**

Neuropathological Changes in Normal Aging, Mild Cognitive Impairment, and Alzheimer's Disease

TERESA GÓMEZ-ISLA
BRADLEY T. HYMAN

From a clinical perspective, Alzheimer's disease has a stereotyped progression, starting with early impairments dominated by memory dysfunction and later evolving into a more generalized dementia with impairments of language, judgment, and executive function. The major structural abnormalities that are believed to be responsible for these impairments are the presence of neurofibrillary tangles and senile plaques and the loss of neurons and synapses. The exact relationship among these lesions, and which of them is most directly responsible for cognitive impairment, remain controversial. Controversy also exists about whether aging and Alzheimer's disease represent a continuum or are dichotomous. Because the progression of cognitive impairment toward dementia of the Alzheimer's disease type is gradual, the idea of an intermediate or transitional stage between healthy aging and dementia of the Alzheimer's disease type has recently gained increasing attention. Whether this transitional stage, which has received several descriptors, including *mild cognitive impairment* (MCI), truly represents the prodromal or earliest clinical phases of Alzheimer's disease dementia is currently under investigation, and studies are underway to precisely define its neuropathological substrate. In this chapter, we will review our experience in studying neuropathological alterations that occur in normal aging, in individuals with very mild cognitive changes, and in persons with Alzheimer's disease. Our data suggest that normal aging is distinct from the neuropathology of mild impairments or of Alzheimer's disease, but that the latter two are remarkably similar in type and neuroanatomical distribution of lesions and are primarily differentiated by the quantity of lesions. Thus many individuals with MCI may well have prodromal Alzheimer's disease from a neuropathological perspective.

We examined in detail a series of individuals who had been given cognitive testing and were known to be either cognitively normal or to have mild dementia (Clinical Dementia Rating [CDR] = 0.5) or severe dementia (CDR = 3.0) prior to death. We previously reported a marked loss of neurons, especially in layer II, in the entorhinal cortex of mildly impaired individuals (Gómez-Isla et al., 1996). We also examined the superior temporal sulcus area of these same individuals to determine the relative degree of neuronal loss and other neuropathological features in a high order association cortex early in the clinical course of Alzheimer's disease.

We studied a total of 81 individuals, 54 of whom had the clinical and neuropathological diagnosis of Alzheimer's disease and 27 of whom were controls. These individuals represent a collection of case material from the Alzheimer Disease Research Center Brain Banks at the Massachusetts General Hospital, at Washington University, and at the Alzheimer's Disease Registry at the Mayo Clinic. The exact methods of clinical evaluation differed slightly among sites and are detailed in our previous publications (Gómez-Isla et al., 1996, 1997). In brief, at the Mayo Clinic and Washington University, the CDR scale was used; at Massachusetts General Hospital, the Blessed Dementia Scale was used. Duration of illness was recorded at all sites. Most important for the analyses highlighted in this report, eight of the cases of Alzheimer's disease fell in the CDR = 0.5 and were clinically very mild or questionable Alzheimer's disease (Table 9–1), whereas the remainder of the Alzheimer's disease cases were at more advanced stages of disease, ranging from moderate to quite severe. The duration of illness ranged from 1 year to over 20 years.

Table 9–1. Cases with a Clinical Dementia Rating (CDR) Scale Score of 0.5 within 1 Year of Death

Gender	Age (years)	Age at onset (years)	Duration (years)	Neuropathological diagnosis
F	95	94	1	Definite AD
M	86	84	2	Definite AD
F	95	94	1	Definite AD
M	85	84	1	Definite AD
M	85	85	0.4	Possible AD
F	81	81	<1	CERAD 1B, 7A
F	94	92	2	CERAD 1B, 6A, 6B
F	91	87	4	CERAD 1B

AD, Alzheimer's disease; CERAD, Consortium to Establish a Registry for Alzheimer's Disease.

The major goal of this study was to examine whether the entorhinal cortex (a major component of the hippocampal neural system related to memory) and the superior temporal sulcus area (a high order association cortex with widespread cortical and limbic connections) developed neurofibrillary tangles, amyloid plaques, and neuronal loss at the same rate over the course of the illness. The temporal lobe was blocked from each of the cases and cut on a freezing microtome in 40 or 50 μ thick sections. The amyloid burden was determined using Aβ immunostaining (antibody 10D5) and a Bioquant image analysis system (Hyman et al., 1992).

Neurofibrillary tangles were visualized using antibody PHF-1 courtesy of Dr Peter Davies (Vincent and Davies, 1992). Neuronal counts and counts of PHF-1-positive neurofibrillary tangles were carried out using stereologically based and statistically unbiased methods, as previously described (Gómez-Isla et al., 1996, 1997). In brief, the volume of the region of interest (either entorhinal cortex or superior temporal sulcus area) was measured using the Bioquant image analysis system for a single 50 μ thick section at a predetermined location. Because of the medial-lateral heterogeneity of the entorhinal cortex sections, the entire breadth of the entorhinal cortex was then assessed in counting chambers selected by using the systematic random counting rule.

The superior temporal sulcus area shows less heterogeneity from medial to lateral but a good deal of heterogeneity from pial surface to white matter junction. The superior temporal sulcus area was assessed using a different strategy, direct counting of contiguous counting chambers from the pial surface to the gray matter–white matter junction in a 700 μ wide region approximately 1 cm from the crown of the middle temporal gyrus in the lower back of the superior temporal sulcus. The optical dissector technique was employed for all counts. Coefficients of error using these methods were below 5%.

The entorhinal cortex occupies the anterior portion of the parahippocampal gyrus and lies adjacent to the amygdala and the uncal hippocampus. Our previous studies examined the entire length of the entorhinal cortex from anterior to posterior (Gómez-Isla et al., 1996). We concluded from that analysis, however, that examination of a section in the center of the entorhinal cortex provided representative data, and the results shown here are derived from examination of a section at the level of the mamillary bodies. Similarly, the superior temporal sulcus region has a good deal of heterogeneity in its far anterior and far posterior extent, and yet is comparable across brains in the center of this anatomical region. We used a section at the level of the lateral geniculate for examination of the superior temporal sulcus area.

We found that, in cognitively normal individuals, there were no changes in either total number of neurons in the entorhinal cortex or superior temporal sulcus area with increasing age, at least over the age range from 60 to 90. This suggests that neuronal loss is not a concomitant of normal aging in these cortical regions. Even within the most vulnerable subareas of these regions (e.g., layer II of the entorhinal cortex) no loss could be detected.

By contrast, in very mild Alzheimer's disease, a marked and statistically significant loss of neurons in entorhinal cortex was observed (Table 9-1). These individuals fit into the CDR = 0.5 category (very mild or questionable impairment). All of these individuals had sufficient neurofibrillary tangles and senile plaques to meet the neuropathological criteria for diagnosis of Alzheimer's disease; neuronal counts in the entorhinal cortex showed a rather dramatic 32% loss compared to the nondemented controls. When we evaluated individual laminae, the results were even more robust. Layer II of entorhinal cortex, perhaps the most vulnerable region in the Alzheimer brain, had about 60% fewer neurons than control cases even in the very mildly impaired individuals. The loss of neurons in entorhinal cortex increased with increasing dementia, reaching 90% in layer II and 70% overall in advanced dementia. This result matches well with the idea that changes in medial-temporal lobe structures and in hippocampus-related neuronal systems are responsible for the early impairments in learning and memory observed at the earliest onset of Alzheimer's disease.

We then examined these same cases for changes in the superior temporal sulcus area. We hypothesized that this high order association cortex would serve neuronal systems related to cognitive systems such as language, face recognition, and the like. As such, we anticipated that in the mildest cases, there may not be changes, but that changes would accrue with increasing duration or severity of dementia. Our data are in accord with this hypothesis. In terms of number of neurons, the CDR = 0.5 cases had a very mild and not statistically significant difference from nondemented controls (Fig. 9–1). However, after a 3 year

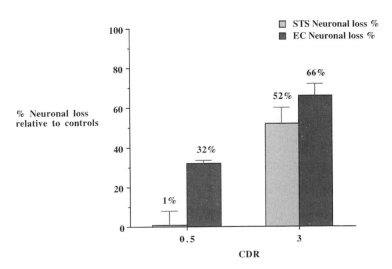

Figure 9–1. Neuronal counts in entorhinal cortex (EC) and superior temporal sulcus area (STS) in very mild Alzheimer's disease (CDR 0.5) relative to severe Alzheimer's disease (CDR 3).

history of dementia, or when patients reach the CDR = 1 (mild dementia) stage, neurons in the superior temporal sulcus (STS) region begin to drop out. Surprisingly, this neuronal loss is linear, with a loss of 7% to 10% per year over this time, until it reaches a maximum of about 70%. This suggests that a substantial subpopulation of neurons, even in highly vulnerable regions, is resistant to Alzheimer's disease–induced loss. A good deal of data point to the relative vulnerability of projection neurons and resistance of interneurons in the neocortex, consistent with sparing of a subpopulation of neurons.

NEUROFIBRILLARY TANGLES AND AMYLOID DEPOSITION

We also examined the number of neurofibrillary tangles and the amount of Aβ deposition in these two cortical areas. The number of neurofibrillary tangles in both areas also correlated well with the duration of illness and the severity of cognitive impairments; by contrast, the amount of immunodetectable Aβ deposits was unrelated to the severity of illness. In other words, individuals with mild disease could have a marked amount of amyloid or just a little; individuals with severe illness could also vary in the amount of amyloid, from comparatively little to marked deposition. In our study of entorhinal cortex (Gómez-Isla et al., 1996), we also assessed the number of PHF tau immunoreactive plaques. The number correlated well with the number of neurofibrillary tangles but not with the total amount of Aβ. Thus, both neurofibrillary tangles and PHF tau containing neuritic plaques correlate with each other and with clinical information. Our most recent studies suggest that neuritic plaques disrupt the neuropil, causing a loss of dendritic structures within their boundaries and thus directly affecting the functional integrity of neural projections in their vicinity (Knowles et al., 1999).

We were interested to learn how these two classic markers of Alzheimer neuropathology would relate to neuronal loss. The stereological methods we used allowed us to perform "checkbook accounting" to ask further questions about the relationship of neurofibrillary tangles and the degree of neuronal loss. We had anticipated that there might be additional neuronal loss that could not be accounted for by neurofibrillary tangle formation. As might be expected from the results presented in the previous paragraph, neurofibrillary tangles were closely correlated with the amount of neuronal loss; for example: $R = .66$, $P < .01$ (Gómez-Isla et al., 1997). However, quantitative analysis showed that neuronal loss was far in excess of the number of neurofibrillary tangles observed. Our data suggest that the ratio of neuronal loss to neurofibrillary tangle formation may be as high as 10 to 1 (Gómez-Isla et al., 1997). By contrast, the percentage of cortex covered by Aβ (amyloid burden) showed no relationship at all to the amount of neuronal loss ($R = .03$, nonsignificant). It may be, however, that a subset of plaques, which are thioflavine S positive, are associated with a local loss of neurons (Urbanc et al., unpublished results).

Thus, although the exact relationships among Aβ deposits, tangle formation, and neuronal loss is not fully defined, it appears that the presence of tangles (and perhaps a subset of plaques) is the tip of the iceberg in terms of marking locations where there has been a great deal of neuronal loss. If true, this suggests that even modest numbers of tangles (e.g., numbers insufficient to meet the neuropathological criteria for Alzheimer's disease) may represent neuronal losses that impact neural system function and hence cognition.

Recent studies suggest that these quantitative measures of Alzheimer-related changes are robust and consistent across several populations. Evaluation of individuals in the Religious Orders Study with mild cognitive impairment revealed a 36% loss of layer II entorhinal cortex neurons compared to controls (Kordower et al., 2001), corresponding to the presence of increased parahippocampal neurofibrillary tangles and neuropil threads (Mitchell et al., 2002). Analogous changes are observed in hippocampal CA1 and the subiculum (Rossler et al., 2002), which lead to changes in hippocampal volume as well (Gosche et al., 2002). Taken together, the data support a continuum of changes that are initially too subtle for clinical detection, followed by an intermediate MCI syndrome, followed by more marked symptoms diagnosed as Alzheimer's disease. It is important to note, however, that there may be substantial person-to-person variability in the exact clinical consequences of some neuropathological changes, and the aging brain in some individuals may be able to maintain normal cognitive function with varying amounts of Alzheimer-like neuropathological changes (Schmitt et al., 2000).

NEURONAL LOSS AS A PROXIMATE CAUSE OF DEMENTIA

Which of the neuropathological changes in the Alzheimer brain cause dementia? Which changes occur earliest? Addressing these issues depends to a great extent on the techniques used to assess the neuropathological changes. In principle, the neuropathological changes of Alzheimer's disease can be differentiated into two categories: positive phenomena such as the formation of senile plaques and neurofibrillary tangles and negative phenomena such as synaptic or neuronal loss. The first are much easier to study for the rather apparent reason that one is examining what can acutally be seen in the Alzheimer brain. Thus qualitative descriptions of senile plaque and neurofibrillary tangle distributions in the cortex appeared soon after the initial report of Alzheimer's disease, and even formal topographic evaluations have been available for over 25 years (Brun and Gustafson, 1976).

By contrast, quantitative studies of neuronal loss are technically more demanding for several reasons. First, because of atrophy, neuronal density does not change as dramatically as one might expect, and it would be fairly easy to miss even substantial changes of 25% or so. Second, a few darkly stained tangles or plaques stand out against a lighter background with silver stains or immunohistochemistry, but loss of a few neurons would not be noticed. Third, inherent in the concept of *loss* is the idea that one can reliably estimate how many neurons existed to start with, and this is difficult, if not impossible, to determine without a substantial group of nondemented individuals. Because of these difficulties, stereological counts on multiple brains are required to assess whether loss has taken place or if the count falls into the normal range. Thus the studies presented here represent some of the first attempts to ask whether neuronal loss matches up, in a quantitative sense, with the presence of neurofibrillary tangles or senile plaques. We find that, at least in the areas studied, neuronal loss matches up much more closely with neurofibrillary tangles.

Our earlier studies of the entorhinal cortex and the superior temporal sulcus area, using different patient populations, suggested that in early Alzheimer's disease there is a substantial number of neurofibrillary tangles, along with marked neuronal loss and relatively few amyloid deposits in entorhinal cortex, whereas in the superior temporal sulcus there are relatively few tangles, mild neuronal loss, and more substantial Aβ (Gómez-Isla et al., 1996, 1997; Hyman, 1997). We have now extended these observations by measuring the entorhinal cortex and superior temporal sulcus in the same cases that had been cognitively assessed during life. These data are in accord with expectations based on the pattern of neurofibrillary tangle development but not of amyloid deposition. Our data show that marked neuronal loss occurs in entorhinal cortex even in cases of mild cognitive impairment, leading to disruption of this neural system. This model is consistent with the idea that cognition is not (detectably) impaired in preclinical Alzheimer's disease in individuals who have some stigmata of Alzheimer-related neuropathology but undetectable amounts of neuronal loss in entorhinal cortex (Price et al., 2001), suggesting that Alzheimer's disease–related neuronal loss is the proximate cause of memory impairment in MCI and in Alzheimer's disease itself.

CLINICAL–PATHOLOGICAL CORRELATIONS: NEURAL SYSTEM DISRUPTION IN LIMBIC AND ASSOCIATION CORTICES

Anatomically, the entorhinal cortex serves as a gateway for projections from sensory-specific and multimodal association cortices to the hippocampus via the perforant pathway, as well as receiving major projections from the hippocampus and initiating feedback projections toward the association cortices. Disruption of these connections would therefore lead to disconnection of the hippocampal formation and the association cortices and thereby would contribute to memory impairment. These data are consistent with an overall scheme of topography of Alzheimer neuropathological changes that is consistent with the most common clinical presentations of the illness (Arnold et al., 1991). Thus, at the earliest point in the disease process, medial temporal lobe structures (including the entorhinal cortex) appear to be affected. Later on, as clinical symptoms representing a broader picture of dementia occur, high order association cortices in the superior temporal sulcus and other neocortical association areas develop changes. Regions such as the superior temporal sulcus area contribute to higher order cognitive functions, including language, integration of sensory afferents, and some aspects of attention. The development of Alzheimer neuropathological changes and neuronal loss later in the disease process therefore likely reflects the clinical observations that symptoms in these cognitive domains frequently occur after the stage of minimal cognitive impairment and are symptoms associated with the clinical diagnosis of Alzheimer's disease.

These data reinforce the previous conclusion that memory loss stems from neuronal depopulation of the entorhinal cortex and related limbic structures and are in accord with expectations based on the pattern of neurofibrillary tangle development (Arnold et al., 1991; Braak and Braak, 1991). Recent data suggest that loss of synaptophysin mRNA occurs in tangle-bearing neurons in the hippocampus as well (Callahan et al., 2002), supporting the overall hypothesis that cortical connectivity is destroyed by a combination of loss of neurons, loss of synaptic integrity (Masliah et al., 2001) and neurofibrillary tangle and neuritic plaque–related changes in the neurophil (Knowles et al., 1999).

RELATIONSHIP BETWEEN ALZHEIMER'S DISEASE AND AGING

Controversy still exists about whether or not aging and Alzheimer's disease should be considered a neuropathological continuum or are dichotomous. Neurofibrillary tangles and senile plaques, the two chief neuropathological hallmarks of Alzheimer's disease, are reported to occur frequently in aging brains. Neurofibrillary tangles are nearly universal in the hippocampal and parahippocampal areas of nondemented individuals over the age of 60 years (Arriagada et al., 1992), and the number increases with age (Braak and Braak, 1991). Numerous diffuse plaques also may be present in many clinically followed nondemented individuals (Delaere et al., 1990; Morris et al., 1996). Furthermore, the distribution of neurofibrillary tangles and senile plaques in various brain regions in the elderly matches the pattern of hierarchical vulnerability seen in Alzheimer's disease and Down's syndrome. However, in our experience, there is no significant age-related neuronal loss in areas that are vulnerable to Alzheimer's disease, including the entorhinal cortex and STS, among carefully followed cognitively intact people (Gómez-Isla et al., 1996, 1997). Clinical studies also suggest that in truly healthy aging people, intellectual performance remains unimpaired over time, whereas sustained decline of even modest proportions may represent a pathological condition (Morris et al., 1991). Our studies suggest, therefore, that Alzheimer's disease is associated with specific neuropathological features including hierarchical vulnerability of limbic and association cortices to neurofibrillary tangles, senile plaques, and neuronal loss and that these changes represent a disease process that, albeit age-related, is independent of normal aging.

NEUROPATHOLOGY AND IMAGING

These data provide the neuropathological and anatomical support for assessing characteristic changes early in Alzheimer's disease by either structural or functional neuroimaging studies. For example, recent data highlight the loss of medial temporal lobe structures in mild Alzheimer's disease (Jack et al., 1997), and quantitative evaluations of the medial temporal lobe structures have proven to be useful in differentiating individuals with mild impairments who progress to dementia from those who do not (Killiany et al., 2000; Dickerson et al., 2001).

SUMMARY

There is evidence that the degenerative process that characterizes Alzheimer's disease may begin many years before the actual clinical diagnosis (Snowdon et al., 1996). The progression of cognitive impairment toward dementia of the Alzheimer's disease type is gradual, and the idea that there is probably an intermediate or transitional stage between healthy aging and dementia of the Alzheimer's disease type has recently become very popular (Petersen, 1995). This transitional stage has received several descriptors such as *mild cognitive impairment* (MCI), *incipient dementia, isolated memory impairment,* and so on. It can be defined as a mild deficit in one or more cognitive domains, but not of sufficient magnitude to constitute the diagnosis of dementia. Whether and how often MCI truly represents the prodromal or earliest clinical phase of Alzheimer's disease dementia is currently the subject of many research efforts, and further studies are necessary to precisely define its neuropathological substrate. However, our current studies suggest that in many instances early memory impairments are associated with specific Alzheimer-related neuropathological changes in limbic areas, which appear to be an early stage of the disease process that ultimately manifests as Alzheimer's disease. Whether or not there is significant neuronal loss in selected memory-related structures of brains with MCI that account for the functional impairment (as we have shown is the case in the entorhinal cortex of dementia patients with very mild Alzheimer's disease) now needs to be clarified. From a practical perspective, the identification of the earliest markers of dementia and Alzheimer's disease progression will allow early interventions in the disease process when therapy might still be effective.

Acknowledgments

This research was supported by National Institutes of Health Grants AG08487 and AG05134 and the Massachusetts Alzheimer's Disease Research Center Brain Bank (Dr. E.T. Hedley-Whyte, director). The clinical and pathological materials are from Washington University's Alzheimer's Disease Research Center (courtesy of Drs. Leonard Berg, John Morris, Dan McKeel, and Joel Price) and the Mayo Clinic Alzheimer Disease Center (courtesy of Drs. Ronald Petersen and Joseph Parisi).

References

Arnold, S.E., B.T. Hyman, J. Flory, A.R. Damasio, and G.W. Van Hoesen. (1991). The topographical and neuroanatomical distribution of neurofibrillary tangles and neuritic plaques in cerebral cortex of patients with Alzheimer's disease. *Cerebral Cortex* 1:103–116.

Arriagada, P.V., K. Marzloff, and B.T. Hyman. (1992). Distribution of Alzheimer-type pathological changes in nondemented elderly matches the pattern in Alzheimer's disease. *Neurology* 42:1681–1688.

Braak, H., and E. Braak. (1991). Neuropathological staging of Alzheimer related changes. *Acta Neuropathol* 82:239–259.

Brun, A., and L. Gustafson. (1976). Distribution of cerebral degeneration in Alzheimer's disease. *Arch Psychiatr Nervenk* 223:15–33.

Callahan, L.M., W.A. Vaules, and P.D. Coleman. (2002). Progressive reduction of synaptophysin message in single neurons in Alzheimer disease. *J Neuropath Exp Neurol* 61:384–395.

Delaere, P., C. Duyckaerts, and C. Masters. (1990). Large amounts of neocortical beta A4 deposits without neuritic plaques or tangles in a psychometrically assessed, non-demented person. *Neurosci Lett* 166:87–93.

Dickerson, B.C., I. Goncharova, M.P. Sullivan, C. Forchett, R.S. Wilson, D.A. Bennett, L.A. Beckett, and L. de Toledo-Morrell. (2001). MRI-derived entorhinal and hippocampal atrophy in incipient and very mild Alzheimer's disease. *Neurobiol Aging* 22:747–754.

Gómez-Isla, T., R. Hollister, H.L. West, et al. (1997). Neuronal loss parallels but exceeds tangle formation in Alzheimer's disease. *Ann Neurol* 41: 17–24.

Gómez-Isla, T., J. Price, D. McKeel, J. Morris, J. Growdon, and B. Hyman. (1996). Profound loss of layer II entorhinal cortex neurons occurs in very mild Alzheimer's disease. *J Neurosci* 16:4991–5000.

Gosche, K.M., J.A. Mortimer, C.D. Smith, W.R. Markesbery, and D.A. Snowdon. (2002). Hippocampal volume as an index of Alzheimer neuropathology: findings from the Nun Study. *Neurology* 58:1476–1482.

Hyman, B.T. (1997). The neuropathological diagnosis of Alzheimer's disease: clinical-pathological studies. *Neurobiol Aging* 18s4:S27–S32.

Hyman, B.T., R.E. Tanzi, K.M. Marzloff, R. Barbour, and D. Schenk. (1992). Kunitz protease inhibitor containing amyloid precursor protein immunoreactivity in Alzheimer's disease: a quantitative study. *J Neuropath Exp Neurol* 51:76–83.

Jack, C.R., Jr., R.C. Petersen, Y.C. Xu, S.C. Waring, P.C. O'Brien, E.G. Tangalos, G.E. Smith, R.J. Ivnik, and E. Kokmen. (1997). Medial temporal atrophy on MRI in normal aging and very mild Alzheimer's disease. *Neurology* 49:786–794.

Killiany, R.J., T. Gómez-Isla, M. Moss, R. Kikinis, T. Sandor, F. Jolesz, R. Tanzi, K. Jones, B.T. Hyman, and M.S. Albert. (2000). Use of structural magnetic resonance imaging in predicting who will get Alzheimer's disease. *Ann Neurol* 47:430–439.

Knowles, R.B., C. Wyart, S.V. Buldyrev, L. Cruz, B. Urbanc, M.E. Hasselmo, H.E. Stanley, and B.T. Hyman. (1999). Plaque-induced neurite abnormalities: implications for disruption of neural networks in Alzheimer's disease. *Proc Natl Acad Sci USA* 96:5274–5279.

Kordower, J.H., Y.P. Chu, G.T. Stebbins, S.T. DeKosky, E.J. Cochran, D. Bennett, and E.J. Mufson. (2001). Loss and atrophy of layer II entorhinal cortex neurons in elderly people with mild cognitive impairment. *Ann Neurol* 49:202–213.

Masliah, E., M. Mallory, M. Alford, R. DeTeresa, L.A. Hansen, D.W. McKeel, Jr., and J.C. Morris. (2001). Altered expression of synaptic proteins occurs early during progression of Alzheimer's disease. *Neurology* 56: 127–129.

Mitchell, T.W., E.J. Mufson, J.A. Schneider, E.J. Cochran, J. Nissanov, L.Y. Han, J.L. Bienias, V.M.Y. Lee, J.Q. Trojanowski, D.A. Bennett, and S.E. Arnold. (2001). Parahippocampal tau pathology in healthy aging, mild cognitive impairment, and early Alzheimer's disease. *Ann Neurol* 51: 182–189.

Morris, J.C., D.W. McKell, Jr., N.I. Storandt, E.H. Rubin, J.L. Price, E.A. Grant, M.J. Ball, and L. Berg. (1991). Very mild Alzheimer's disease: informant-based clinical, psychometric, and pathologic distinction from normal aging. *Neurology* 41:469–478.

Petersen, R.C. (1995). Normal aging, mild cognitive impairment, and early Alzheimer's disease. *Neurologist* 12:326–344.

Price, J.L., A.I. Ko, M.J. Wade, S.K. Tsou, D.W. McKell, and J.C. Morris. (2001). Neuron number in the entorhinal cortex and CA1 in preclinical Alzheimer disease. *Arch Neurol* 58:1395–1402.

Rossler, M., R. Zarsi, J. Bohl, and T.G. Ohm. (2002). Stage-dependent and sector-specific neuronal loss in hippocampus during Alzheimer's disease. *Acta Neuropathol* 103:363–369.

Schmitt, F.A., D.G. Davis, D.R. Wekstein, C.D. Smith, J.W. Ashford, and W.R. Markesbery. (2000). "Preclinical" Alzheimer disease revisited: neuropathology of cognitively normal older adults. *Neurology* 55:370–376.

Snowdon, D.A., S.J. Kemper, J.A. Mortimer, L.H. Greiner, D.R. Wekstein, and W.R. Markesbery. (1996). Linguistic ability in early life and cognitive function and Alzheimer's disease in late life: findings from the nun study. *JAMA* 275:528–532.

Vincent, I., and P. Davies. (1992). A protein kinase associated with paired helical filaments in Alzheimer's disease. *Proc Natl Acad Sci USA* 89:2878–2882.

CHAPTER **10**

Biological Markers

NEILL R. GRAFF-RADFORD

Alzheimer's disease (AD) is the commonest cause of dementia, affecting more than four million Americans over the age of 65 years and with an estimated cost to the United States of $100 billion per year (Small et al., 1997). Unless an effective treatment is found, the cost is likely to increase, particularly when the "baby boomers" reach the risk age period. The ideal treatment strategy is to identify those at risk and prevent their developing the disease. An accurate diagnostic marker would be helpful because clinical diagnosis is only about 85% accurate (Small et al., 1997). Further, when we find markers related to AD, we must ask how these findings relate to the biology of the disease. The better our understanding of the disease, the greater our chances of combating it. Markers that help monitor the effects of treatment or direct appropriate treatments to the subpopulations also would be useful.

VALUES OF MARKERS

In summary, the value of finding markers for AD include:

1. Increasing the accuracy of clinical diagnosis
2. Identifying those at risk

3. Understanding the biology
4. Monitoring progression of disease and effect of treatment and selecting populations in whom treatment is effective

Making an Accurate Diagnosis

For point one, making an accurate diagnosis, we should know the following for any marker:

- Sensitivity—true positive / true positive + false negative
- Specificity—true negative / true negative + false positive
- Positive predictive value—true positive / true positive + false positive
- negative predictive value—true negative / true negative + false negative
- Prior probability—true positive + false negative / total population

At present, sensitivity and specificity studies are difficult to perform. One major problem is that AD is a chronic disease so that determining if the patient has or is free of disease at one point in time might be misleading; for example, controls scoring normally on neuropsychological tests could be developing AD pathology but not have reached the threshold where cognition is affected. In such cases, a marker may give an apparent false positive but actually portend the development of AD. Further, autopsy patients who don't quite meet the pathological criteria for AD might show indications of developing the disease. In such cases, too, the marker may be thought to give a false positive result.

There is no gold standard against which we can measure marker accuracy. If we measure against the clinical diagnosis of probable AD, we know the clinical diagnosis is only about 85% accurate, compared to pathological diagnosis. This is one of the reasons that the Consensus Report of the Working Group on Molecular and Biochemical Markers (1998) recommends that markers be validated against neuropathologically confirmed cases. However, the pathological diagnosis also varies, depending on which criteria are used. The new pathological guidelines for the diagnosis of AD (Consensus Recommendations for the Post-mortem Diagnosis of Alzheimer's Disease, 1997) still have to be validated. One way around this difficulty is by comparing markers to continuous pathological variables, such as the number and distribution of tangles, a quantification of different types of plaques and the amount of cell loss, rather than arbitrary cut scores of pathological findings. The new pathological criteria, which quantify both tangle and plaque pathology, would lend themselves to this approach. Another important confound when evaluating markers is the overlap of AD and other pathological diagnoses such as vascular dementia (VD) and diffuse Lewy body disease (DLB). Depending on the way these data are handled, overlapping cases could be classified as falsely positive or negative. In the initial studies of a marker, perhaps overlapping cases should be analyzed separately.

We believe that these are some of the compelling reasons that researchers evaluating markers should do longitudinal studies, ideally from the presymptomatic stage through the evolution of the disease and to autopsy.

Identifying Persons at Risk

Regarding point two, that is, identifying persons at risk, we already know that possessing specific mutations on the amyloid precursor protein (APP) in the presenilin-1 and presenilin-2 genes predicts AD at a specific age range. Other risk factors are increasing age, a family history of dementia, and having one or more apolipoprotein E (APOE)-4 genes.

Investigators evaluating markers that could predict AD should do longitudinal studies that depend on detecting incident cases of AD developing in the population being followed. However, we know that only 1% of individuals older than age 65 years develop AD per year. This means that researchers would have to follow 1000 persons for 1 year to find 10 cases of AD. To carry out such a study in an unselected population would be very expensive because the investigators would have to follow a very large cohort for a prolonged period.

Researchers can use certain strategies to increase the incident cases in a given population, however. The first is studying an older population because the incidence of AD increases with age. Kokmen and colleagues (1988) showed that the incidence of AD is about 66/100,000 per year for people age 60 to 69 years; 409/100,000 per year for people age 70 to 79 years; and 1479/

100,000 per year for people older than age 80 years, so a smaller elderly cohort could be followed to obtain the same number of incident cases in a given time. Using this strategy has the disadvantage that earlier onset AD cases may have different risk factors to later onset cases—for example, the known FAD mutations occur early and *APOE-4* shifts the onset of AD to an earlier age. Another strategy to enrich the cohort with incident cases is to choose first-degree AD relatives in whom the AD risk is higher (Mortimer, 1995) than that of the general population. The disadvantage of this strategy is that it selects for genetic factors and an effective marker may not apply to sporadic cases. By combining these two strategies—that is, follow first-degree relatives of AD patients older than 65—a more manageable and less expensive initial longitudinal study can be undertaken.

Understanding the Biology

Point three, understanding the biology of AD by identifying disease markers, is a crucial strategy to move the field forward. Excellent examples already exist and include knowing that:

- There are genetic markers such as APP, presenilin-1 and presenilin-2 mutations
- Apolipoprototein E genotype changes the risk
- In all early-onset familial forms of AD (FAD), Aβ42 is increased in the plasma
- Tau protein is increased in the cerebrospinal fluid (CSF) of AD patients

It is clear that these discoveries have had a major effect on the AD field.

Monitoring Progression

Point four, monitoring progression and effect of treatment and selecting populations in whom treatment is effective, is important, and a few examples exist. Some studies indicate that patients with AD and apolipoprotein E4 may not improve as well with acetylcholine esterase inhibitors; however, other reports dispute this (Farlow et al., 1998) Nonetheless, it would be a distinct advantage if by using certain markers we are able to identify subpopulations in whom medication is effective. In monitoring AD treatment it would be useful to have a marker that measures the amount of pathology, the evolution of pathology over time, and the treatment effects on pathology in vivo. Examples of this could include a radioisotope measure of the amount of amyloid in the brain, magnetic resonance imaging (MRI) measures of volume loss of certain brain structures such as the hippocampus, MR spectroscopy measuring biochemical changes in the brain, increasing CSF tau, changing plasma or CSF $A\beta$ levels, evolving APP isoforms in platelets, changing measures of inflammation in the blood (perhaps the p97 protein), and evolving psychometric test scores. For the evaluation of treatments such as immunization against $A\beta42$ (Schenk et al., 1999) and medication that inhibits the secretases crucial in $A\beta$ formation (Vassar et al., 1999), monitoring markers such as plasma and CSF $A\beta$ levels may be particularly important.

The Consensus Report of the Working Group on Molecular and Biochemical Markers of Alzheimer's Disease (1998) proposed that a diagnostic marker for AD should have as many of the following features as possible:

- Able to detect a fundamental feature of Alzheimer's neuro-pathology
- Validated in neuropathologically confirmed cases
- Precise (able to detect AD early in its course and distinguish it from other dementias)
- Reliable
- Noninvasive
- Simple to perform
- Inexpensive

In this chapter we discuss in some detail five markers for AD:

1. CSF tau
2. Plasma and CSF $A\beta$ levels
3. Platelet APP protein isoforms
4. The iron binding protein p97
5. Neural thread protein

We have chosen these because we think that they have the most promise at present. Other chapters in this book discuss the FAD genes and apolipoprotein E4.

TAU IN THE CSF

One of the observations Alzheimer made in the first case he described, which was later named after him, was that there were silver staining abnormalities in neurons (Alzheimer, 1907). These neurofibrillary tangles have a similar structure to the neuropil threads and dystrophic neurites also found in AD. (For a review see Trojanowski et al., 1996). They are composed of paired helical filaments (PHFs), which, in turn, have been found to be mainly composed of the microtubule-associated protein tau in abnormally phosphorylated forms. Tau is a phosphoprotein that binds to and promotes the stability of microtubule-associated protein (MAP) at three or four highly conserved repeat regions. It consists of six alternatively spliced proteins encoded by the same gene on chromosome 17. Tau is important in a number of neurodegenerative diseases—for example, 95% of PSP patients have a polymorphism on exon 10 of the tau protein compared to the same polymorphism seen in only 55% of controls (Conrad et al., 1997).

A Western blot of Alzheimer's brain shows three major bands, called "triplet paired helical filament tau" by Dickson (1997). Other diseases with triplet paired helical filament tau are Down syndrome, postencephalitic Parkinsonism, Guam Parkinson dementia complex, and familial NFT-only dementia. Immunoblots of tau in other diseases with tau inclusions show only two bands and have what is termed "doublet PHF-tau." This group includes Pick disease, PSP, CBD, and FTDP-17 dementia (Dickson 1997).

An important recent report showed that missense and 5'-splice mutations in the tau gene cause frontotemporal dementia and parkinsonism (Hutton et al., 1998). Some of these mutations increase the four-repeat compared to the three-repeat forms of tau. Most important, these findings demonstrate that tau dysfunction can lead to neurodegeneration.

With this as background, it is interesting to evaluate the numerous studies measuring tau in the CSF of patients with AD. Table 10–1 summarizes many of these reports.

A number of important points emerge when we evaluate these studies:

1. The studies consistently show higher levels of tau in the CSF of AD patients than in normal controls.
2. CSF tau levels increase early in AD. In one study (Andreason et al., 1999b), 205 AD patients with a Mini-Mental State Examination (MMSE) score of >23, the CSF tau level was 653 ± 321pg/ml, and the sensitivity of detecting these patients was 193 out of 205, or 94%.
3. CSF tau is increased in at least one genetic form of AD—in symptomatic and presymptomatic patients with the APP 670/671 mutation.
4. There are important false negatives (AD patients with normal levels) and false positives (other dementia patients such as FTD, DLB, VAD, CJD, NPH, CPA, and less often PSP and CBD; see Table 10–1 for abbreviations). Of less diagnostic significance, tau is increased in the CSF of other neurological diseases such as ALS, neuropathy, stroke, and inflammatory diseases.
5. There is no consistent correlation with severity of disease (inverse correlation in three reports, but no correlation in eight reports).
6. One study (Tapiola et al., 1998) showed that the levels of CSF tau increased with *APOE-4* gene dosage, but in another this was not seen (Andreason et al., 1999b).
7. CSF tau levels had low interindividual variation on repeated sampling at a 1-year interval (Andreason, 1999b). There is a strong correlation between the CSF tau levels measured 1 year apart, in probable AD $r = .64$ ($p < .00001$) and possible AD $r = .75$, $p < .00001$.

It is possible that as the biology is better understood and more specific tau antibodies are raised—such as the one reported by Itoh and colleagues (2001) against tau protein phosphorylated at serine 199 (in which the sensitivity was 85.2% and the specificity 85% for AD ($n = 236$) against a large group of non-AD-demented and nondemented patients ($n = 239$)—this test may improve in accuracy. An important drawback is the need for lumbar puncture to do this test. Significant increase of ac-

Table 10–1. Reports of tau in the Cerebrospinal Fluid (CSF) of Patients with Alzheimer's Disease

Study/year	AD	Normals	Neurological diseases	Other dementias	Significant difference AD/NC	Comments
Vandermeeren et al., 1993	27	51	129	Included in the 129	Yes	False +ve, degen. diseases, inflam, stroke
Blennow et al., 1995	44	31	15	Vas (17) FLD (11)	Yes	False +ve, VAD, FLD, PD
Nitsch, 1995	19					τ did not correlate with severity
Tato et al., 1995	23	23		36	Yes	Inverse correlation with MMSE, positive correlation with glucose, VAD higher than controls but lower than AD
Vigo-Pelfrey et al., 1995	71	26	59	25	Yes	False +ve, FTD, VAD, ALS, neuropathy, no correlation with MMSE
Munroe et al., 1995	24	14	26		Yes	False +ve in 3 NC, 1 Binswanger's and 1 depression, no correlation with MMSE
Jensen et al., 1995	21	22	31		Yes	Tau increased in 6 with 670/671 APP (pre and symptomatic) mutation, no correlation with MMSE
Rosler et al., 1996	16	37			Yes	Inverse correlation with MMSE
Hock et al., 1995	19	18	20		Yes	Inverse correlation with MMSE
Arai et al., 1995, 1998	70/97	19/15	96/59	(see 1997)	Yes	False +ve, stroke, AIDS, inflam.
Arai, 1997				FTD (8), PSP (6), CBD (3), DLB (6)		More overlap with AD of FTD and DLB than PSP and CBD
Galasko, 1997	36	14	10	9	Yes	Increased tau seen in early AD. No correlation with MMSE

Study						Comments
Kanai et al., 1998	93	54	56	33	Yes	Tau increases on repeat LP, there is a correlation with MMSE
Galasko et al., 1998	82	60		74	Yes	False +ve in FTD, VAD, CPA, PDD, LBD, depression, MCI, lyme disease, NPH. No correlation with MMSE
Tapiola et al., 1998	81		33	43	No normal controls	CSF tau more increased with ApoE 4 gene dosage
Andreason et al., 1999b	407	65	28 with depression		Yes	Sensitivity 93% and specificity of 86% compared to controls. 193 had f/u LP at 1 year and tau stable. High in early AD, level not related to severity
Hulstaert et al., 1999	150	100	84	79	Yes	This is a multicenter study. False +ve for FTD, VAD, NPH and other degenerative dementias. At 85% sensitivity specificity was 58%
Kahle et al., 2000	30	16	29 PD without dementia	DLB (5)	Yes	No correlation with MMSE. An autopsy proved 'pure LB' case had an increased tau level
Itoh et al., 2001	236	95	122	FTD (16), PSP (21), CBD (15), LBD (13), VAD (23), CjD (11), INFLAM (18)	Yes	Antibody to phosphorylated τ at serine 199. Sensitivity 85.2% and specificity 85%. False +ve in FTD, CBD, PSP, DLB, VAD and CjD

Abbreviations: AD (Alzheimer's disease), CBD (corticobasal dementia), DLB (dementia with Lewy bodies), FTD (frontotemporal dementia), PSP (progressive supranuclear palsy), CPA (chronic progressive aphasia), VAD (vascular dementia), PDD (Parkinson disease dementia), mild cognitive impairment (MCI), NPH (normal pressure hydrocephalus), NC (normal controls), Inflam (inflammatory neurological diseases), ALS (amyotrophic Lateral Sclerosis), MMSE (Mini Mental State Examination), APP (Amyloid Precursor Protein).

curacy over clinical diagnosis would have to occur to make this a routine diagnostic test.

Aβ40 AND Aβ42

The amyloid precursor protein (βAPP) is coded on chromosome 21 and is a 690 to 770 amino acid transmembrane protein with a carboxyl (COOH) end inside the cell and an amino (NH2) end outside the cell. The amino acids are numbered from the amino (NH2) end. In the longest form of the βAPP (770 amino acids), 1 to 699 are outside the cell, 700 to 723 are in the membrane, and 724 to 770 are inside the cell. There are two main pathways of metabolism:

1. There is a proteolytic cleavage after amino acid 687 by an unknown protease called α secretase, followed by cleavage at 711 or 713 amino acid (apparently in the membrane) by an enzyme called γ secretase (which may be presenilin-1).
2. There is proteolytic cleavage after amino acid 671 by a recently identified enzyme β secretase (Vassar et al., 1999), followed by cleavage at 711 or 713 amino acid (in the membrane) by γ secretase.

Pathway two results in the production of Aβ1-40 and Aβ1-42 species, which are normally secreted. For review, see Selkoe (1996).

Secreted Aβ is readily detected in cerebrospinal fluid, in plasma, and in the medium in which a wide variety of cultured cells are grown. In each of these situations, most secreted Aβ is Aβ1-40, but a small component (5% to 10%) is Aβ1-42. Aβ ending at 42 is especially important in AD. Aβ1-42 forms amyloid fibrils in vitro much more rapidly than does Aβ1-40, and there is excellent evidence that Aβ42 is deposited early and selectively in senile plaques. (For review, see Younkin 1995.) It is for these reasons that Aβ has been studied as a marker for AD.

Aβ IN CSF

There are numerous studies supporting that there are lower levels of Aβ42 in the CSF of AD patients. A summary of some of these studies follows.

Aβ1-42 levels in CSF were compared between patients with AD ($n = 37$), normal controls ($n = 20$), and neurological controls ($n = 32$). As a group the AD patients had significantly lower levels than either control group ($p < .0001$); however, there was much overlap between the groups. A cutoff of 505 pg/ml best separated AD patients from the other groups. No AD patient had a level below 505 pg/ml, giving a sensitivity of 100%, and 33 of 52 controls had levels above 505 pg/ml, giving a specificity of 63%. There was no significant correlation between the level and age or sex and MMSE score. Aβ1-42 levels in CSF were not influenced by the APOE genotype (Motter et al., 1995).

Tamoaka and colleagues (1997) reported the CSF Aβ1-42(3), AβX-42(3), Aβ1-40, and AβX-40 levels in 20 sporadic AD patients and 34 neurological controls. In the AD patients, there were significantly lower Aβ1-42(3) and AβX-42(3) levels than in controls ($p < .01$) but no significant difference between groups in the Aβ1-40 and AβX-40 levels. The ratio of AβX-42(3) to Aβ1-42(3) was significantly increased in the AD patients ($p < .05$). They conclude that the ratio of amino terminal truncations and modifications of CSF Aβ42(3) with carboxy termini ending at the residue 42(3) was higher in the AD group than in the controls. Possible explanations of the lower levels of Aβ42(3) in the CSF of AD patients include greater adsorption to amyloid deposition, lower secretion, and higher clearance from CSF (Tamaoka et al., 1997).

Kanai and colleagues (1998) reported Aβ40 and Aβ42 CSF levels in 93 AD patients (32 followed longitudinally with repeat CSF levels), 33 non-AD patients, 56 patients with other neurological diseases, and 54 normal controls. They also measured CSF tau simultaneously. There was a significant decrease in Aβ42 and an increase in the ratio of Aβ40 to Aβ42 in AD patients over those in the controls. The longitudinal study showed continuous low Aβ42 and an increase in the ratio of Aβ40 to Aβ42 before the onset of AD. Kanai et al. (1998) devised an AD index of tau CSF levels multiplied by Aβ40/Aβ42. This index gave the best sensitivity (71%) and specificity (83%) in the cross-sectional patients. In the longitudinal patients, this index increased the sensitivity to 91%.

Galasko and colleagues (1998) measured Aβ42 and tau in the CSF of 82 patients with AD, 60 cognitively normal (NC) elderly controls, and 74 subjects with other causes for dementia (ND). Aβ42 was significantly lower and levels of tau were significantly higher in the AD group than in the NC and ND groups. In the AD group, Aβ42 levels were inversely associated with *ApoE-4* allele dosage and weakly related to the MMSE. Combining CSF Aβ42 and tau levels, the tests were 90% sensitive and 80% specific in distinguishing normal controls from AD patients. However, using both tests, 26 of 74 ND patients were misclassified as AD patients. So far, 12 of 13 patients who underwent autopsy were correctly classified with the combined CSF tests.

Hulstaert and colleagues (1999) reported the results of a multicenter study evaluating the usefulness of CSF Aβ42 and tau protein as diagnostic tests for AD. There were 150 probable AD patients, 100 healthy volunteers or patients with disorders not associated with pathological conditions of the brain, 84 patients with other neurological disorders, and 79 patients with non-AD dementia. The median CSF Aβ42 level was 487 pg/ml for AD patients, 849 pg/ml for normal controls, 643 pg/ml for neurological disease, and 603 pg/ml for non-AD dementia. All control groups were significantly different from AD ($p < .001$). At 85% sensitivity, specificity of combined Aβ42 and tau tests was 86% (95% CI: 81% to 91%), compared with 55% (95% CI: 47% to 69%) for Aβ42 alone and 65% (95% CI: 58% to 72%) for tau alone. The combined test at 85% sensitivity was 58% (95% CI: 47% to 69%) for non-AD dementia. Interestingly, the *APOE* gene load was negatively correlated with Aβ42 levels in AD and non-AD dementia.

Samuels and colleagues (1999) found that there was a positive correlation between CSF Aβ40 and Aβ42 and MMSE. Further, there was a stronger correlation of CSF Aβ42 and MMSE in those who were APOE-33 homozygotes. From this they postulated that APOE-33 homozygotes may have a different mechanism of Aβ deposition and clearance than patients with different APOE genotypes.

Andreasen and colleagues (1999a) reported on the CSF Aβ42 levels in a 20-month follow-up study in 53 probable AD patients. They found that the CSF Aβ levels were significantly lower in AD patients with 709 ± 304 pg/ml ($n = 53$), compared to controls with 1648 ± 436 pg/ml ($n = 21$) $p < .001$. There was a strong correlation between baseline levels and 1-year follow-up levels (r = .90; p < .001). There was no significant correlation between duration of disease or severity measured by MMSE. Low CSF $A\beta42$ levels were found in those with mild dementia MMSE > 25. Interestingly, those with early-onset AD had significantly lower CSF $A\beta42$ levels (422 ± 170 pg/ml) than those with late-onset (845 ± 255 pg/ml) p < .001.

In contrast to Andreason's study, Tapiola and colleagues (2000) reported a 3-year follow-up study of CSF tau, $A\beta40$, and $A\beta42$ (n = 17). There was a significant reduction of CSF $A\beta42$ with time (p < .05). Concentration decreased in 14 of 17 patients; in those with duration of 2 years or less of disease, the levels decreased even more. $A\beta40$ decreased in 15 of 17 patients (p < .05). CSF tau levels increased in nine and decreased in eight patients.

Otto and colleagues (2000) reported that CSF $A\beta42$ levels were decreased in 27 Creutzfeldt-Jakob disease patients, compared to normal controls (n = 20) and other non-AD dementia patients (n = 19), but there was no significant difference from a group of AD patients (n = 12). This is an important false positive $A\beta42$ test to be taken into account.

Marauyama and colleagues (2001) reported a study showing that MCI patients (n = 19) who all developed AD at follow up (others who did not progress to AD were excluded) had CSF $A\beta42$ levels the same as normal controls. Over time, their $A\beta42$ CSF levels decreased significantly (from 539.5 ± 149.6 pg/ml to 397.6 ± 164.1 pg/ml). They found a significant correlation with the $A\beta42$ level and the MMSE in the AD, MCI, and control groups. This study supports the notion that at the time of MCI the $A\beta42$ levels may be normal, but they decrease as AD develops.

Andreason and colleagues (2001a) reported a study using the combination of $A\beta42$ and tau protein as a diagnostic test in 241 consecutive community-based patients. Other reported studies were in referral medical centers. Higher levels of tau and lower levels of $A\beta42$ in combination gave a diagnostic sensitivity of 94% in probable AD, 88% in possible AD, and 75% in MCI. The presence of an *APOE-4* allele increased the sensitivity to 99% for probable AD (73/74), 100% for possible AD (27/27), and

88% for MCI (7/8). In a primary care setting, as in this study, this test may be useful, but the additive value in a specialty center is yet to be known.

Thus, measuring $A\beta 42$ but not total $A\beta$ in the CSF can be used as a diagnostic marker for AD. As illustrated in the studies by Kanai and colleagues (1998), Galasko and colleagues (1998), and Hulstaert and colleagues (1999), combining $A\beta$ and tau CSF measures increases the diagnostic accuracy. Even in combination, Growden (1998) noted that for the AD index to be accepted as a useful and diagnostic test in early AD, its sensitivity and specificity should be improved. Galasko (1998) noted that autopsy follow-up will be needed to decide whether CSF false positives are true false positives or whether AD is the primary diagnosis in these cases. At this time it is uncertain whether CSF $A\beta$ levels decrease in time, as indicated in by Tapiola and colleagues, or remain stable, as found by Andreason and colleagues. This could be important because serial measures of CSF could be one way of monitoring therapies directed against $A\beta$.

Regarding MCI, the study by Maruyama et al. (2001) indicates that CSF $A\beta 42$ is close to normal in those who develop AD over time, while Anreasen et al. (1999a) show that those with early dementia (MMSE > 25) already have low $A\beta 42$ CSF levels. Further in their community-based study, Andreason et al. (2001b) found 75% sensitivity for diagnosing MCI using both CSF tau and $A\beta 42$ in combination. For diagnostic purposes and monitioring treatment, this is a crucial issue and worthy of further study.

Regarding other dementias, Vanmechelen and colleagues (2001) summarized this subject. In Lewy body dementia, recent studies have shown a decrease in CSF $A\beta 42$ with a normal tau level. Those with frontotemporal dementia (FTD) often (in about half the cases) have an increase in CSF tau (not as high as AD) but normal $A\beta 42$. Patients with Creutzfeld-Jakob disease have very high CSF tau levels and lower $A\beta 42$ levels, showing that deposition is probably not the only mechanism of having a reduced level of CSF $A\beta 42$.

$A\beta$ IN PLASMA

In a series of studies we have measured plasma $A\beta 40$ and $A\beta 42$ and found the following:

- Levels of Aβ40 and Aβ42 are significantly higher in late-onset AD patients than in age-matched controls, and plasma Aβ levels decrease with duration and severity of disease (Graff-Radford et al., 2000). Mehta and colleagues (2000) also found that Aβ40 (but not Aβ42) plasma levels are higher in AD patients than in controls.
- Aβ42 is higher in patients with all the early-onset genetic forms of AD—that is, those with mutations on APP, presenilin-1, and presenilin-2 (Scheuner et al., 1996).
- Aβ40 and Aβ42 increase with age, starting at 65 years (Graff-Radford et al., 1996).
- Aβ40 and Aβ42 are higher than in age-matched controls in Down syndrome patients starting in the first decade (Graff-Radford et al., 1997).
- Aβ42 is increased in more than 25% of presymptomatic first-degree relatives of AD patients compared to only 7% of matched controls (Graff-Radford et al., 1998).
- We identified first degree relatives, younger than 65 years, of AD patients. Then we measured their plasma Aβ levels and identified those with high levels. With the proband in this group, we then collected blood specimens from five extended families and found that Aβ levels were higher in members of the families across three generations. Also, as a group, these extended families had higher plasma levels than controls and the married-in members of the families. (Graff-Radford et al., 1998).

All of these findings have led us to the following hypotheses:

1. Extracellular Aβ increases because of (*a*) known genetic factors (mutations on APP, presenilin-1, presenilin-2, and Down syndrome); (*b*) unknown genetic factors (25% of relatives with AD have increased plasma Aβ levels, and this is genetically determined as indicated by these increased levels being seen across three generations in five extended families), and we have plasma Aβ42 to find a locus on chromosome 10 that is related to late-onset Alzheimer's disease (Ertekin Taner et al., 2000); and (*c*) increasing age (passed age 65 years).
2. The higher extracellular Aβ levels can be measured in the plasma.

3. As Aβ is deposited in the brain, there is a decrease in extracellular measures of Aβ as noted by (*a*) the decrease in CSF
Aβ levels in patients with AD; (*b*) the decrease in plasma Aβ
levels with increasing duration of disease; and (*c*) the decrease
of plasma levels in the Hsiao transgenic mice as they deposit
Aβ in their brains (unpublished data).

To study the implications of high plasma Aβ levels, a longitudinal study is essential because in cross-sectional studies patients have conflicting influences on the plasma levels; for instance, age and genetic factors increase the levels, while
deposition of Aβ decreases levels. Mayeux and colleagues (1999)
completed such a study. They followed a group of normal elderly
individuals in Manhattan and had plasma stored at the beginning
of the study. After an average follow-up of 3.6 years, 105 were
still normal but 64 had converted to probable AD or incipient
AD (a clinical dementia rating [CDR] scale of 1 or 0.5, respectively.) They found a significant difference in plasma Aβ40, Aβ42,
and the ratio of Aβ42 to Aβ40 between the two groups. In a
multivariate analysis adjusting for age, education, APOE genotype, and ethnic group, Aβ42 (but not Aβ40) remained significantly different. Some 50% percent of patients in the upper quartile of Aβ42 levels developed AD, compared to 8% in the lowest
quartile. While this study should be replicated in other populations and by other investigators, it does raise hope that part of
the risk of developing AD may be predicted by measuring plasma
Aβ levels.

How increased Aβ and the presence of one or two *APOE-4*
genes interact is yet to be determined. In presymptomatic relatives of AD patients who are homozygous for the *APOE-4* allele
($n = 11$), the plasma levels were significantly lower than age-
matched *APOE-33* homozygotes (Graff-Radford et al., 1998). Because this is cross- sectional data, at least two possibilities may
explain the finding. Either the plasma levels in the *APOE-44* homozygotes had already decreased when the individuals were studied, or *APOE-44* leads to Aβ brain deposition at a time before
extracellular Aβ is increased.

We suggest that plasma Aβ may be a promising marker that
could predict some of the risk of developing AD. We believe that
additional longitudinal studies are essential to test this hypothe-

sis. We also believe that yet unidentified genetic factors are important in the pathogenesis of late-onset AD and that plasma $A\beta$ may be useful in monitoring treatments that affect $A\beta$, such as immunization against $A\beta 42$ and drugs that inhibit β and γ secretases.

AMYLOID PRECURSOR PROTEIN ISOFORMS IN PLATELETS

Di Luca and colleagues (1998) summarized the different APP isoforms found in platelets as follows:

> Three major APP isoforms are present in membranes of resting platelets and both platelets and megakaryocytes express 3 APP transcripts encoding for APP 695, APP 751 and APP 770. Activated platelets release membrane fragments containing the mature full length APP751/770 and the carboxyl truncated form of APP stored in alpha granules (protein nexin II).

They reported that the longer APP form (130 kd) decreased in AD and with severity of AD and that the ratio of the longer to the shorter (110 and 106 kd) APP isoforms was particularly helpful in differentiating AD from normal controls and non-AD dementia. There was a significant difference between AD patients ($n = 32$), normal controls ($n = 25$), and non-Alzheimer's disease dementia ($n = 16$) ($p < .01$). They have now extended this finding to include mild AD and MCI patients (Padovani et al., 2002). They compared 35 patients with mild AD, 21 with very mild AD, and 30 MCI patients to 25 age-matched controls. The APP platelet forms ratio (APPr) was significantly decreased in patients with mild AD (0.44 ± 2.4; $p < 0.001$), very mild AD (0.49 ± 0.3; $p < 0.001$), and MCI (0.62 ± 0.33; $p < 0.002$). Fixing the cutoff score at 0.6, sensitivity was 88% for patients with mild AD, 86% for very mild AD, and 60% for MCI. While this test has some very promising features such as being a blood test, it also has some drawbacks. Patients on medication that affects platelet function have to be off the medication for at least 2 weeks. Medications include anticholinergic, antiplatelet agents, serotoninergic medications, anticoagulants, and steroids. Drawing the blood for harvesting platelets is complicated. Nonetheless, this test is certainly worthy of further study. Others have confirmed the AD finding (Rosenberg, 1997).

NEURONAL THREAD PROTEIN

The neural thread proteins (NTP) are a family of proteins expressed in the brain and immunologically related to pancreatic thread protein. In 1992, de la Monte and colleagues reported that at autopsy the brains of AD patients contained more neural thread protein immunoreactivity than did control brains (de la Monte and Wands, 1992) and that, in the CSF, levels of NTP were increased in advanced AD cases, correlating with progression of dementia (de la Monte et al., 1992).

In 1997, de la Monte and colleagues reported that they had isolated cDNA, which they called AD7c-NTP. It is expressed in neurons and overexpressed in AD. Using an enzyme-linked sandwich immunoassay, they detected a recombinant protein with a molecular mass of 41 kD in the CSF of 323 clinical and postmortem patients. They found that the concentration of this protein in ventricular postmortem CSF in 121 AD patients (9.2 ± 8.2 ng/ml) was significantly higher than in 19 aged controls (1.6 ± 0.0 ng/ml) $p < .0001$. In clinical patients, the concentration in the lumbar CSF in 89 probable and possible AD patients (4.6 ± 3.4 ng/ml) was higher than in 18 controls (1.2 ± 0.07 ng/ml), in 32 Parkinson's disease patients (1.8 ± 1.1 ng/ml), and in 41 multiple sclerosis patients (1 ± 0.9 ng/ml) $p < .0001$. In the clinical AD sample, the concentration of the protein increased significantly with the Blessed Dementia Scale Score ($p < .0001$) but not with age. Levels of above 3 ng/ml identified 62% of patients with the clinical diagnosis of AD and 84% of pathological AD cases.

This same group (Ghanbari et al., 1998) has studied AD7C-NTP in urine as an AD marker. They found that in an AD group of 66 and a non-AD group of 134, there was a significant difference in the urine levels of the neural thread protein.

In a recent essay, Kahle and colleagues (2000) reported a study in which neuronal thread protein levels were measured in the CSF of 35 demented patients (25 with probable AD, 5 with definite AD at autopsy, and 5 with Lewy body pathology at autopsy) and were compared to 29 nondemented Parkinson's patients and 16 healthy elderly controls. Levels of neuronal thread protein were significantly higher in AD patients than in the controls; the sensitivity was 70% and the specificity was 87% in distinguishing nondemented controls from AD patients. Neuronal thread protein had a small but significant inverse correlation with MMSE ($r = -0.43$).

As can be seen, this is a diagnostic marker that warrants further study. Further proof that it meets criteria for a good diagnostic marker remains to be shown, particularly with validation by several independent groups.

p97

So far there has only been one article on this subject, describing p97 as a marker in AD (Kennard et al., 1996). The iron binding protein, p97, also known as melanotransferrin, belongs to the family of iron binding proteins, including transferrin, lactoferrin, and ovotransferrin. There are two forms of p97, one attached to cell surface by glycosyl-phosphatidylinositol and the other actively secreted. p97 is highly localized to capillary endothelium cells of human brain. p97 is specifically expressed on reactive microglial cells associated with amyloid plaques in postmortem brain tissue from AD patients. The serum p97 levels in 17 AD patients was 43.8 ± 11.6 ng/ml and in 15 normals 7.04 ± 3.28 ng/ml. There was a significant difference between groups ($p = 6.6 \times 10^{-10}$) and no overlap of levels in patients and normals. There was also a significant increase of p97 serum levels with length of disease. In the CSF of five AD patients, the mean p97 levels were 22.4 ± 9.21, compared to a mean of 8.48 ± 4.02 ng/ml in five controls with other neurological diseases. This was significantly different ($p < .05$).

An abstract reporting, a larger series (AD, $n = 35$; controls, $n = 64$) at the international Alzheimer's meeting in Amsterdam continues to show a significant difference in p97 levels between AD patients and controls (Jefferies et al., 1998). The serum p97 was measured in 35 consecutive AD patients with possible or probable AD and compared to 64 control patients. As a group, the AD patient p97 levels were twice as high as those in the control group. The AD patients' levels were bimodal for uncertain reasons.

These are very early interesting reports and meet the criteria of being noninvasive and possibly simple to perform and inexpensive. The other criteria for a diagnostic marker still have to be shown. We await future studies with interest.

CONCLUSION

At this time, there is no universally accepted biological marker for Alzheimer's disease. The five markers discussed have promise and with additional refinement may become clinically useful. From the point of view of improving diagnostic accuracy of AD CSF tau, CSF Aβ42, and APP isoforms in platelets, neural thread protein and p97 may become useful. To monitor treatments directed against Aβ, plasma and CSF Aβ levels would be important to monitor but any of the above markers would be of interest. To predict future risk of developing AD, plasma Aβ has some promise.

Acknowledgments

This work is supported in part by P50 AG16574 and AG06656.

References

Alzheimer, A. (1907). Über eine eigenartige Erkrankung der Hirnrinde. *Allg Zt Pschiatrie psychisch-Gerichtliche Med (Berlin)* 64:146–148.

Andreason, N., C. Hesse, P. Davidson, L. Minthon, A. Wallin, B. Winblad, et al. (1999a). Cerebrospinal fluid β-amyloid (1–42) in Alzheimer's disease. *Arch Neurol* 56:673–680.

Andreason, N., L. Minthon, et al. (1999b). Sensitivity, specificity, and stability of CSF-tau in AD in a community-based patient sample. *Neurology* 53:1488–1494.

Andreason, N., J. Gottfries, et al. (2001a). Evaluation of CSF biomarkers for the axonal and neuronal degeneration, gliosis, and β-amyloid metabolism in Alzheimer's disease. *J. Neurol Neurosurg Psychiatry* 71:557–558.

Andreason, N., L. Minthon, et al. (2001b). Evaluation of CSF-tau and CSF-Aβ42 as diagnostic markers for Alzheimer disease in clinical practice. *Arch Neurol* 58:373–379.

Arai, H., M. Terajima, et al. (1995). Tau in cerebrospinal fluid: a potential diagnositc marker in Alzheimer's disease. *Ann Neurol* 38(4):649–652.

Arai, H., C. Clark, et al. (1998). Cerebrospinal fluid Tau protein as a potential diagnostic marker in Alzheimer's disease. *Neurobiol Aging* 19: 125–126.

Blennow, K., A. Wallin, et al. (1995). Tau protein in cerebrospinal fluid: a biochemical marker for axonal degeneration in Alzheimer disease? *Mol Chem Neuropathol* 26(3):231–245.

Conrad, C., A. Andreadis, et al. (1997). Genetic evidence for the involvement of τ in progressive supranuclear palsy. *Ann Neurol* 41:277–281.

Consensus Recommendations for the Postmortem Diagnosis of Alzheimer's Disease. (1997). *Neurobiol Aging* 18(S4):S1–S2.

Consensus Report of the Working Group on Molecular and Biochemical Markers of Alzheimer's Disease. (1998). *Neurobiol Aging* 19:109–116.

de la Monte, S., and J. Wands. (1992). Neuronal thread protein overexpression in brains with Alzheimer's disease lesions. *J Neurol Sci* 113:153–164.

de la Monte, S., L. Volicer, et al. (1992). Increased levels of neuronal thread protein in cerebrospinal fluid of patients with Alzheimer's disease. *Ann Neurol* 32:733–742.

de la Monte, S., K. Ghanbari, et al. (1997). Characterization of the AD7C-NTP cDNA expression in Alzheimer's disease and measurement of a 42-kD protein in the cerebrospinal fluid. *J Clin Invest* 100:3093–3104.

Dickson, D. (1997). Neurodegenerative diseases with cytoskeletal pathology: a biochemical classification. *Ann Neurol* 42:541–544.

Di Luca, M., L. Pastorino, et al. (1998). Differential levels of platelet amyloid β precursor protein isoforms. *Arch Neurol* 55:1195–1200.

Ertekin Taner, N., N. Graff-Radford, et al. (2000). Linkage of plasma Aβ42 to a quantitative locus on chromosome 10 in late-onset Alzheimer's disease pedigrees. *Science* 290:2303–2304.

Farlow, M., D. Lahiri, et al. (1998a). Metrifonate in the symptomatic treatment of Alzheimer's disease: influence of apolipoprotein E genotype. *Neurology* 50:(S4)A88.

Farlow, M., D. Lahiri, et al. (1998b). Outcome of tacrine depends on apolipoprotein genotype and subject gender. *Neurologue* 50:669–677.

Galasko, D., C. Clark., et al. (1997). Assessment of CSF levels of tau protein in mildly demented patients with Alzheimer's disease. *Neurology* 48:632–635.

Galasko, D., L. Chang, et al. (1998). High cerebrospinal fluid tau and low amyloid β42 levels in the clinical diagnosis of Alzheimer's disease and relation to Apolioprotein E genotype. *Arch Neurol* 55:937–945.

Ghanbari, H., K. Ghanbari, et al. (1998). Biochemcial assay for AD7C-NTP in urine as an Alzheimer's disease marker. *J Clin Lab Anal* 12:285–288.

Graff-Radford, N., C. Eckman, et al. (1996). Amyloid β protein in plasma of Alzheimer's disease patients and controls. *Neurology* 46:A161.

Graff-Radford, N., C. Eckman, et al. (1997). Plasma amyloid β protein (Aβ) in Down's syndrome (DS): implications for Alzheimer's disease. *Neurology* 47:A378.

Graff-Radford, N., C. Eckman, et al. (1998). Plasma amyloid (Aβ) levels in relatives of Alzeimer's disease patients. *Neurology* 48:A314.

Graff-Radford, N., L. Younkin, et al. Plasma Aβ levels are increased in Alzheimer's disease and decrease with progression. *Neurololgy* 54S3:A316.

Growden J. (1998). To tap or not to tap: cerebrospinal fluid markers of Alzheimer's disease. *Ann Neurol* 44:6–7.

Hock, C., S. Golombowski et al. (1995). Increased levels of tau protein in cerebrospinal fluid of patients with Alzheimer's disease: correlation with degree of cognitive impairment [letter]. *Ann Neurol* 37(3):414–415.

Hulstaert, F., K. Blennow, et al. (1999). Improved discrimination of AD patients using β-amyloid(1–42) and tau levels in CSF. *Neurologue* 52: 1555–1562.

Hutton, M., C. Landon, et al. (1998). Association of missence and 5′-splice mutations in tau with the inherrited dementia FTDP-17. *Nature* 393: 702–705.

Itoh, N., H. Arai, et al. (2001). Large-scale, multicenter study of cerebrospinal fluid tau protein phophorylated at serine 199 for the antemortem diagnosis of Alzheimer's disease. *Ann Neurol* 50:150–156.

Jefferies, W., H. Feldman, et al. Serum p97 as a screening test for Alzheimer's disease. *Neurobiol Aging* 19(4S):S82.

Jensen, M., H. Basun, et al. (1995). Increased cerebrospinal fluid tau in patients with Alzheimer's disease. *Neurosci Lett* 186(2–3):189–191.

Kahle, P., M. Jakowec, et al. (2000). Combined assessment of tau and neuronal thread protein in Alzheimer's disease CSF. *Neurology* 54:1498–1504.

Kanai, M., E. Matsubara, et al. (1998). Longitudinal study of cerebrospinal fluid levels of tau, Aβ1-40, and Aβ1-42(3) in Alzheimer's disease: a study in Japan. *Ann Neurol* 44:17–26.

Kennard, M., H. Feldman et al. (1996). Serum levels of the iron binding protein p97 are elevated in Alzheimer's disease. *Nat Med* 2:1230–1235.

Kokmen, E., V. Chandra, et al. (1988). Trends in incidence of dementing illness in Rochester, Minnesota, in quinquennial periods, 1960–1974. *Neurology* 38:975–980.

Maruyama, M., H. Arai, et al. (2001). Cerebrospinal fluid amyloid β1-42 levels in the mild cognitive impairment stage of Alzheimer's disease. *Exp Neurol* 172:433–436.

Mayeux, R., M.-X. Tang M-X, et al. Plasma amyloid β-peptide 1-42 and insipient Alzheimer's disease. *Ann Neurol* 46:412–416.

Mehta, P., T. Pirttila et al. Plasma and cerebrospinal fluid levels of amyloid β proteins 1-40 and 1-42 in Alzheimer's disease. *Arch Neurol* 57:100–105.

Mortimer, J.A. (1995). The epidemiology of Alzheimer's disease: beyond risk factors. In *Research Advances in Alzheimer's Disease and Associated Disorders*, edited by I. Iqbal, J. Mortimer, B. Winblad, and H. Wisniewski (pp. 3–13). New York: John Wiley and Sons.

Motter, R., C. Vigo-Pelfrey, et al. (1995). Reduction of β-amyloid peptide 42 in the cerebrospinal fluid of patients with Alzheimer's disease. *Ann Neurol* 38(4):643–648.

Munroe, W.A., P.C. Southwick, et al. (1995). Tau protein in cerebrospinal fluid as an aid in the diagnosis of Alzheimer's disease. *Ann Clin Lab Sci* 25(3):207–217.

Nitsch, R.M., G.W. Rebeck, et al. (1995). Cerebrospinal fluid levels of amyloid β protein in Alzheimer's disease: inverse correlation with severity of dementia and effect of apolipoprotein E genotype. *Ann Neurol* 37: 512–518.

Otto, M., H. Esselman, et al. (2000). Decreased β-amyloid 1-42 in cerebrospinal fluid of patients with Creutzfeldt-Jakob disease. *Neurology* 54: 1099–1102.

Padovani, A., B. Borroni, et al. (2002). Abnormalities in the pattern of platelet amyloid precursor protein forms in patients with mild cognitive impairment and Alzheimer's disease. *Arch Neurol* 59:71–75.

Rosenberg R.N., F. Baskin, et al. (1997). Altered amyloid protein processing in platelets of patients with Alzheimer's disease. *Arch Neurol* 54:139–144.

Rosler, N., I. Wichart, et al. (1996). Total tau protein immunoreactivity in lumbar cerebrospinal fluid of patients with Alzheimer's disease. *J Neurol Neurosurg Psychiatry* 60:237–238.

Samuels, S., J. Silverman, et al. (1999). CSF β-amyloid, cognition, and *APOE* genotype in Alzheimer's disease. *Neurology* 52:547–551.

Schenk, D., R. Barbour, et al. (1999). Immunization with amyloid-β attenuates Alzheimer-disease-like pathology in the PDAPP mouse. *Nature* 400:173–177.

Scheuner, D., C. Eckman, et al. (1996). Aβ42(43) is increased in vivo by the PS1/2 and APP mutations linked to familial Alzheimer's disease. *Nat Med* 2:864–870.

Selkoe, D. (1996). Amyloid β-protein and the genetics of Alzheimer's disease. *J Biol Chem* 271:18295–18298.

Small, G., V. Rabins, et al. (1997). Diagnosis and treatment of Alzheimer's disease and related disorders: consensus statement of the American Association for Geriatric Psychiatry, the Alzheimer's Association and the American Geriatric Society. *JAMA* 278:1363–1371.

Tamaoka, A., N. Sawamuara, et al. (1997). Amyloid β protein 42(43) in cerebrospinal fluid of patients with Alzheimer's disease. *J Neurol Sci* 148: 41–45.

Tapiola, T., M. Lehtovirta, et al. (1998). CSF tau is related to apolipoprotein E genotype in early Alzheimer's disease. *Neurology* 50:169–174.

Tapiola, T., T. Pirttila, et al. Three year follow-up of cerebrospinal fluid tau, β-amyloid 42 and 40 concentrations in Alzheimer's disease. *Neurosci Lett* 280:119–122.

Tato, R., A. Frank, et al. (1995). Tau protein concentrations in cerebrospinal fluid of patients with dementia of the Alzheimer's type. *J. Neurol Neurosurg Psychiatry* 59:280–283.

Trojanowski, J., C. Clark, et al. (1996). Elevated levels of tau in cerebrospinal fluid: implications for the antemortem diagnosis of Alzheimer's disease. *Alzheimer's Disease Rev* 1:77–83.

Vandermeeren, M., M. Merken, et al. (1993). Detection of tau proteins in normal and Alzheimer's disease cerebrospinal fluid with sensitive sandwich enzyme-linked immunosorbent assay. *J Neurochem* 61:1828–1834.

Vanmechelen, E., H. Vanderstichele, et al. (2001). Cerebrospinal fluid τ and β-amyloid 1-42 in dementia disorders. *Mechanisms Ageing Development* 122:2005–2011.

Vassar, R., B. Bennett, et al. (1999). Secretase cleavage of Alzheimer's amyloid precursor protein by the transmembrane aspartase protease BACE. *Science* 286:735–740.

Vigo-Pelfrey, C., P. Seubert, et al. (1995). Elevation of microtubule-associated protein tau in the cerebrospinal fluid of patients with Alzheimer's disease. *Neurology* 45:788–793.

Younkin, S. (1995). Evidence that Aβ42(3) is the real culprit in Alzheimer's disease. *Ann Neurol* 37:287–288.

CHAPTER **11**

Clinical Evaluation

RONALD C. PETERSEN

When a person presents with a memory complaint or an informant suspects a memory problem, the clinician must decide if this complaint warrants a thorough evaluation. If a cognitive complaint is a major concern for the subject, then an evaluation should be undertaken. The clinical evaluation of a person with a suspected memory problem is similar to that of a dementia evaluation (Petersen, 2003). Presuming that we are discussing the amnestic form of a mild cognitive impairment (MCI), the primary history and evaluation should revolve around issues of memory performance.

HISTORY

The history from the patient and informant is a critical element in assessing the nature of the problem. The history should focus on the recall of recent events. Since remote memories may be preserved in a mild memory disorder, the history should emphasize the recall of events that have occurred in recent days or weeks. One approach involves asking the patient questions about current events or significant items in the news in recent weeks or months. This type of information can include information

about natural disasters, crimes, or items concerning political figures. It is important to assess the likelihood with which the subject would have been exposed to this type of information. If the
person reads a daily newspaper, watches the news on television,
or monitors current events on the radio, these questions become
legitimate. However, if the individual is rarely exposed to these
types of information, this line of questioning would be inappro-
priate. If the subject happens to be a sports fan, one can pursue
this line of questioning to draw on the subject's personal interests. For example, if the subject were a professional football fan,
one could ask questions about the person's favorite team and its
recent fate. If there are particularly noteworthy players, one
could inquire about their recent performances.

This line of questioning is not quantitative but can give the
clinician an impression of the person's ability to recall details of
presumably incidentally learned material. If the subject tends to
be somewhat vague about the details of these events, the clinician
can suspect that the memory for these experiences may be somewhat faulty.

The clinician also needs to be aware of the subject's general
cognitive function. The clinician needs to be certain the patient
is not aphasic or inattentive and therefore could be having difficulties with memory secondary to other cognitive problems. Patients and families often attribute all problems in cognition to
memory when, in fact, the deficit may reside in another cognitive
domain.

Occasionally, information can be obtained regarding memory function simply during the interview itself. If the subject has
traveled to the clinician's office, one can ask questions about the
route of travel, method of transportation, and other events of
the past 24 hours. Again, this gives the clinician insight into the
person's ability to recall recently experienced events.

It is often necessary to interview the informant separately.
Occasionally, family members or friends may feel uncomfortable
answering questions about forgetfulness in the presence of the
subject. Therefore, a separate interview inquiring about recently
experienced events may enable the clinician to ask personalized
questions of the subject. It is also important to get the informant's opinion on how the person's memory is functioning currently and how it is functioning relative to the recent past. It is

important to determine a temporal course for the evolution of the memory problem.

NEUROLOGICAL EXAMINATION

Once the histories from the subject and informant are completed, the clinician should perform a complete neurologic examination on the subject. The neurologic examination should include a mental status evaluation.

Mental Status Evaluation

The mental status examination should survey a variety of cognitive domains, including, at a minimum, learning, recall, attention, language, problem solving, executive function, and visuospatial function. There are several standardized instruments for this purpose, such as the Mini-Mental State Exam (Folstein et al., 1975) and the Kokmen Short Test of Mental Status (Kokmen et al., 1991). None of these instruments is perfect however. To be most sensitive for MCI, the instrument should have either features of learning material over a series of trials or a delayed recall component for that material, or both. Often in the brief survey, there is a short list of words presented and recalled after a period of time. The Kokmen Short Test of Mental Status has an advantage over the Mini-Mental State Exam insofar as there are four words to be remembered, and a greater delay filled with intervening activities is interspersed between the learning trials and the recall portion of the exam. In the scoring of the instrument, the number of words learned and the number of words recalled after a delay are all factored into the score. This makes this instrument somewhat more sensitive to early memory changes.

While these instruments have "cutoff scores" that are often cited, such as the score of 24 on the Mini-Mental State Exam and a score of 29 on the Kokmen Short Test of Mental Status, these scores are not to be used in an absolute fashion. In particular, for subjects with MCI, the overall scores might be quite high— Mini-Mental scores in the 25 to 28 range and Kokmen Short Test scores in the 30 to 35 range. A person may have an impairment in memory function but perform well in all of the other cognitive domains. In fact, this would be entirely consistent with the amnestic form of MCI.

In the office setting, memory can be evaluated with more extensive sets of verbal and nonverbal materials. As mentioned, it is important to give a sufficient number of items to be learned such that the subject has to acquire the material over several learning trials. Then, if a delay interval of 15 to 30 minutes can be introduced, recall after that delay can be quite sensitive to the earliest aspects of a memory impairment. Some investigators indicate that the type of processing that is done in learning the materials can be critically important in assessing subsequent recall. Tests such as the Memory Impairment Screen (Buschke et al., 1999) emphasize the semantic processing done during the learning period. This can be a useful measure of memory performance.

A brief memory instrument developed by Knopman and Ryberg (1989) can also be useful in the office setting. Because this test involves semantic processing of a list of words, it can be quite sensitive to early memory impairments.

Weintraub (2000) has emphasized the importance of individualizing the memory task for the subject by proposing a list learning exercise based on the subject's own word span (Weintraub, 2000). This technique ensures that the subject must transfer the information from a temporary store into a more "permanent" store to retain the material (see Figure 11–1). This also

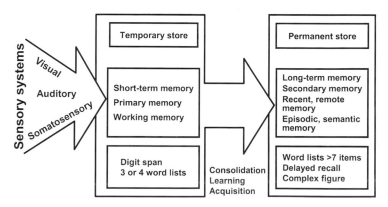

Figure 11–1. Information processing scheme showing flow of information through sensory association areas to a temporary and ultimately to a relatively permanent storage networks. [Reproduced with permission of Churchill Livingston (Petersen, 2003).]

stresses the information-processing network at its most vulnerable point (Petersen, 2003).

As mentioned, the mental status examination should also evaluate other cognitive domains. If a person has a memory impairment, this could be secondary to poor attention or to comprehension or other cognitive difficulties. For example, a patient with an aphasia with a significant anomia may appear to be having difficulties with memory. However, after testing, memory may prove to be quite adequate and the person may have a relatively circumscribed lesion—perhaps in the left anterior temporal lobe—that is producing the profound anomia. Other patterns of performance can be suggestive of certain disorders as well. For example, a relatively flat learning curve on a multiple trial free-recall word list task can indicate poor effort or depression (Petersen, 1991, 2003). This opinion can be reinforced if there is relatively good delayed recall of the amount learned, even though the amount learned is less than one would expect.

Neuropsychological Testing

Neuropsychological testing can be considered as an extension of the mental status examination. In general, the same concerns regarding mental status testing can be carried over into the neuropsychology laboratory. The testing should survey function in multiple cognitive domains. In the case of MCI, the clinician will be primarily interested in the results of the learning and recall measures, as well as in performance in other cognitive domains. Typically, a subject with MCI may have a slightly depressed learning curve, indicating that learning efficiency is not normal. Most important, however, there will be a deficit in delayed recall. For example, if the subject has learned a list of 15 words over five learning trials, delayed recall of that list after 30 minutes of intervening activities may reveal performance that is significantly impaired. If a subject learned 10 of the 15 words by the fifth trial of the learning phase, the subject may only recall 2 after a 30-minute delay. This performance would be indicative of impaired delayed recall, and this can be the earliest sign of a memory impairment (Petersen et al., 1992, 1994; Welsh et al., 1991).

Neuropsychological testing raises questions as to the appropriate standards for comparison (see Chapter 4 and 5). Typically, a subject's performance may be compared to age- and education-matched individuals. These norms may present the most adequate comparison for these subjects, but this comparison standard is somewhat controversial (Ivnik et al., 1991; Sliwinski et al., 1996). Other considerations would include a measure of the subject's prior performance, but this is often not available (Collie et al., 2001). Some investigators have advocated comparing memory performance to the performance of young individuals on the same instruments (Crook et al., 1986). However, research has indicated that, depending on the specific type of memory test employed, this degree of deficit could be observed in virtually all elderly subjects, and the intepretation of this impairment is unclear (Smith et al., 1991).

The shape of the learning curve and the relative degree of delayed recall performance can be useful in discriminating among conditions. As is seen in Figure 11–2, if a subject exhibits a normal learning curve, the person should acquire more words on each learning trial. After a delay of 15 to 30 minutes, most of the material should be recalled. However, in the setting of depression one may find a flattened learning curve with relatively preserved delayed recall. As noted, this may indicate a lack of

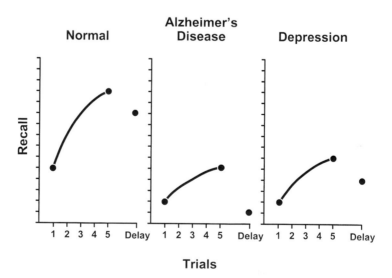

Figure 11–2. Theoretical learning curves depicting normal, depressed, and Alzheimer's disease subjects. [Reproduced with permission of Churchill Livingston (Petersen, 2003).]

effort or attention on the part of the subject secondary to the depression. However, once the material is learned, it is recalled efficiently because the essential neurocognitive mechanisms involved in learning and recall are still intact. In the setting of a degenerative disease such as Alzheimer's disease (AD), the subject may exhibit a depressed learning curve and impaired delayed recall. This may result from disease involving medial temporal lobe structures, which are central for the learning and recall process (Petersen et al., 2000).

The discussion thus far has centered on verbal learning materials. These instruments tend to be more commonly available, and, hence, more research has been conducted with verbal materials. However, it is also possible that a subject may have difficulties with nonverbal materials. Consequently, a thorough neuropsychological exam should involve the learning and recall of nonverbal materials as well since this may reflect disease in the nondominant hemisphere (Lezak, 1995; Weintraub, 2000).

The neuropsychological test battery should assess aspects of attention, language, visuospatial skills, problem solving, praxis, and constructions. Assessment of these domains will help the clinician determine if memory is the sole cognitive function impaired and if it is impaired out of proportion to other cognitive abilities. For the diagnosis of amnestic MCI, it would be important for the clinician to observe a decrease in memory function with relative preservation of the other cognitive domains.

Ultimately, however, in making the diagnosis of MCI, the clinician must exert the final judgment. While neuropsychological testing can be critically important in establishing a cognitive profile and determining the degree of memory impairment, the neuropsychological testing by itself does not make the diagnosis of MCI. The clinician must combine features of the history, mental status exam in the office, and general neurologic and medical exams, along with neuropsychological testing, to make the final diagnostic decision.

GENERAL NEUROLOGICAL EXAMINATION

The clinician should also perform a complete neurological exam to see if there are abnormalities in other areas of function. For example, if the subject exhibited features of rigidity, bradykinesia, or postural imbalance, with or without a tremor, an extrapyramidal disorder can be considered. Parkinson's disease, parkinsonism, or other Lewy body disorders can be present with subtle cognitive impairments early in their evolution. If the subject was found to have a visual field deficit or asymmetric reflexes, mass lesions or vascular insults could be entertained. The asymmetry of the neurologic findings may speak to a disease process other than a degenerative condition. However, the clinician must keep in mind that degenerative conditions can present in an asymmetric fashion as well, and, consequently, the temporal course of the disorder is important. The general neurologic exam can also give clues to etiology. If the subject has features of a prominent peripheral neuropathy, one could entertain possible toxic or metabolic contributions to the change in cognition. The neurological examination can be illuminating with regard to the nature of the underlying disorder.

GENERAL MEDICAL EXAMINATION

The subjects should also be examined from a general medical perspective as well. A prominent sensory deprivation such as cataracts or a severe hearing impairment can affect the patient's cognitive function. An unstable medical condition such as congestive heart failure, poorly controlled diabetes mellitus, or pulmonary conditions can affect cognitive function in a secondary fashion. Consequently, an overall general medical examination should be carried out to determine the subject's overall medical status.

PSYCHIATRIC EXAMINATION

Since cognitive symptoms can be the presenting feature of some psychiatric conditions, these disorders need to be entertained as well. As discussed, depression can present with learning inefficiencies and memory problems. Anxiety can also compromise the subject's ability to remember, and this aspect of the subject's overall condition should be explored. Here again, a complete interview with the subject and an informant can be quite helpful in determining any psychiatric contributions to the cognitive impairment.

NEUROIMAGING

After a patient has been suspected of having a memory impairment and cognitive testing has documented a deficit, neuroimaging studies can be considered. Computed tomography (CT) scans can be adequate for ruling out major structural lesions such as a subdural hematoma, tumor, large infarct, or hydrocephalus. However, magnetic resonance imaging (MRI) scans are preferable with respect to imaging structures that may be involved in isolated memory impairments or subtle cognitive deficits. MRI scans that focus on the temporal lobes, the thalamus, the basal forebrain, and other interconnecting pathways in the limbic system can be particularly useful. Contrast agents can be helpful in bringing out lesions that affect the blood–brain barrier or in visualizing infarctions.

In recent years, neuroimaging of structures germane to memory function have been informative in evaluating MCI. The most advanced studies at this time involve structural imaging of the hippocampus and other medial temporal lobe structures (Jack et al., 1997, 1999). As was discussed in Chapter 6, volumetric imaging of the hippocampus can be particularly useful in delineating structural counterparts to amnestic disorders. For example, in MCI atrophy of the hippocampi are commonly seen and not only can be helpful in the diagnostic phase of the disorder but also can predict or suggest the longitudinal course of subjects with MCI (Jack et al., 1999). Studies of volumetric assessment of the entorhinal cortex have also been helpful, and there is some controversy over the relative usefulness of entorhinal versus hippocampal measurements (Killiany et al., 2000; Xu et al., 2000). It is generally recommended that MRI scans that focus on medial temporal lobe structures should be done in assessing subtle memory disorders.

Structural neuroimaging studies can also be useful in suggesting possible etiologies of the memory impairment. For example, areas of infarction in the limbic system or atrophy suggesting degeneration can be quite useful to the clinician. Most standard MRI facilities are able to provide this information.

FUNCTIONAL NEUROIMAGING

Since these disorders are often subtle and may present as the earliest stages of a more ominous process, functional imaging studies can be useful. While they are relatively less well developed than the structural imaging studies, functional imaging can be informative (Johnson et al., 1998). In particular, with positron emission tomography (PET), areas of hypometabolism can be seen in the posterior cingulate or occasionally in medial temporal lobe regions (Minoshima et al., 1997; Silverman et al., 2001). Some studies have indicated that persons who are at risk for developing AD by virtue of their apolipoprotein E4 status might show areas of hypometabolism in the temporal parietal regions while they are still asymptomatic (Reiman et al., 1996; Small et al., 1995). Finally, magnetic resonance spectroscopy studies are in their relative infancy but have suggested that there may be chemical shift changes that differentiate subjects with MCI from both normal aging and individuals with mild AD (Kantarci et al., 2000).

ELECTROPHYSIOLOGY

Electroencephalograms can be considered in individuals who may have a suggestion of the seizure disorder. Since the hippocampal region of the medial temporal lobe is one of the more epileptogenic regions in the brain, subtle isolated seizure discharges in this region can be disruptive to memory function. While this is an uncommon form of a memory impairment, it should always be considered since it is potentially treatable. Occasionally, a subtle complex partial seizure disorder can present with a memory deficit, and, consequently, an electroencephalogram—ideally with sleep deprivation—can be considered.

LABORATORY EVALUATION

If the history, neurological exam, medical exam, neuropsychological evaluation, and neuroimaging studies suggest a specific etiology, laboratory studies can be oriented in that direction. The temporal course of the memory disorder can be important in helping to determine the nature of the laboratory investigation.

However, if the situation suggests a gradual degenerative condition such as an amnestic form of MCI that may be a harbinger of a degenerative dementia such as AD, laboratory studies that are typically performed for evaluation of a dementia can be considered. These studies are shown in Table 11–1. These studies do not need to be carried out in all cases but can be considered by the clinician. In addition, a cerebrospinal fluid analysis may be considered, as indicated in Table 11–1. As mentioned, the

Table 11–1. Laboratory Studies to be Considered in Evaluation of Memory Problems

Chemistry group
Hematology group
Sedimentation rate
Vitamin B-12 level
Folic acid level
Thyroid function studies
Anti-nuclear antibody
Extractable nuclear antigen
HIV
Lyme serology
Syphilis serology
Toxicology screening
Alcohol level
Copper and ceruloplasmin
Anti-cardiolipin antibodies
Lupus anticoagulant
Paraneoplastic autoantibody panel
Arterial blood gas
Cerebrospinal fluid studies
    Cell count
    Total protein
    Glucose
    Syphilis serology
    IgG index
    IgG synthesis rate
    Oligoclonal bands
    Gram stain
    Cultures for bacteria fungi
    Mycobacteria and viruses
    Polymerase chain reaction for herpes simplex virus or
      B. burgdorferi
    Cytology

temporal course and other medical conditions can dictate which of these studies, if any, need to be considered (Petersen, 2003).

SUMMARY

The evaluation of a suspected memory disorder can be complex. The importance of an accurate history from the patient and a knowledgeable informant cannot be overemphasized. The nature of the memory impairment, if present, can be suggested by temporal course, family history, other medical conditions, and certain lifestyle features of the subject. If the subjects are in their 70s or 80s, the prospect of a degenerative disease becomes much greater. However, the clinician needs to be mindful of unusual presentations of other disorders as well. Memory disorders can be serious and debilitating conditions, and, consequently, a thorough clinical and laboratory evaluation may be warranted.

References

Buschke, H., G. Kuslansky, M. Katz, W.F. Stewart, M. Sliwinski, H.M. Eckholdt, and R.B. Lipton. (1999). Screening for dementia with the Memory Impairment Screen. *Neurology* 52(2):231–238.

Collie, A., P. Maruff, R. Shafiq-Antonacci, M. Smith, M. Hallup, P.R. Schofield, C.L. Masters, and J. Currie. (2001). Memory decline in healthy older people: implications for identifying mild cognitive impairment. *Neurology* 56:1533–1538.

Crook, T., R.T. Bartus, S.H. Ferris, P. Whitehouse, G.D. Cohen, and S. Gershon. (1986). Age-associated memory impairment: proposed diagnostic criteria and measures of clinical change—Report of a National Institute of Mental Health Work Group. *Devel Neuropsychol* 2:261–276.

Folstein, M.F., S.E. Folstein, and P.R. McHugh. (1975). "Mini-Mental State": a practical method for grading the cognitive state of patients for the clinician. *J Psychiatr Res* 12(3):189–198.

Ivnik, R.J., G.E. Smith, E.G. Tangalos, R.C. Petersen, E. Kokmen, and L.T. Kurland. (1991). Wechsler Memory Scale: IQ-dependent norms for persons ages 65 to 97 years. *Psychol Assess* 3:156–161.

Jack, C.R. Jr., R.C. Petersen, Y.C. Xu, S.C. Waring, P.C. O'Brien, E.C. Tangalos, G.E. Smith, R.J. Ivnik, and E. Kokmen. (1997). Medial temporal atrophy on MRI in normal aging and very mild Alzheimer's disease. *Neurology* 49(3):786–794.

Jack, C.R. Jr., R.C. Petersen, Y.C. Xu, P.C. O'Brien, G.E. Smith, R.J. Ivnik, B.F. Boeve, S.C. Waring, E.G. Tangalos, and E. Kokmen. (1999). Prediction of AD with MRI-based hippocampal volume in mild cognitive impairment. *Neurology* 52(7):1397–403.

Johnson, K.A., K.J. Jones, J.A. Becker, A. Satlin, B.L. Holman, and M.S. Albert. (1998). Preclinical prediction of Alzheimer's disease using SPECT. *Neurology* 50:1563–1571.

Kantarci, K., C.R. Jack Jr., Y.C. Xu, N.G. Campeau, P.C. O'Brien, G.E. Smith, R.J. Ivnik, B.F. Boeve, E. Kokmen, E.G. Tangalos, and R.C. Petersen. (2000). Regional metabolic patterns in mild cognitive impairment and Alzheimer's disease: a 1H MRS study. *Neurology* 55(2):210–217.

Killiany, R.J., T. Gomez-Isla, M. Moss, R. Kikinis, T. Sandor, F. Jolesz, R. Tanzi, K. Jones, B.T. Hyman, and M.S. Albert. (2000). Use of structural magnetic resonance imaging to predict who will get Alzheimer's disease. *Ann Neurol* 47:430–439.

Knopman, D.S., and S. Ryberg. (1989). A verbal memory test with high predictive accuracy for dementia of the Alzheimer type. *Arch Neurol* 46: 141–145.

Kokmen, E., G.E. Smith, R.C. Petersen, E. Tangalos, and R.J. Ivnik. (1991). The short test of mental status: correlations with standardized psychometric testing. *Arch Neurol* 48(7):725–728.

Lezak, M.D. (1995). Neuropsychological Assessment, Vol. 3. New York: Oxford University Press.

Minoshima, S., B. Giordani, S. Berent, K.A. Frey, N.L. Foster, and D.E. Kuhl. (1997). Metabolic reduction in the posterior cingulate cortex in very early Alzheimer's disease. *Ann Neurol* 42:85–94.

Petersen, R.C. (1991). Memory assessment at the bedside. In Memory Disorders, edited by T. Yanagihara and R.C. Petersen (pp. 137–152). New York: Dekker.

Petersen, R.C., G. Smith, E. Kokmen, R.J. Ivnik, and E.G. Tangalos. (1992). Memory function in normal aging. *Neurology* 42:396–401.

Petersen, R.C., G.E. Smith, R.J. Ivnik, E. Kokmen, and E.G. Tangalos. (1994). Memory function in very early Alzheimer's disease. *Neurology* 44:867–872.

Petersen, R.C., C.R. Jack Jr., Y.C. Xu, S.C. Waring, P.C. O'Brien, G.E. Smith, R.J. Ivnik, E.G. Tangalos, B.F. Boeve, and E. Kokmen. (2000). Memory and MRI-based hippocampal volumes in aging and AD. *Neurology* 54(3): 581–587.

Petersen, R.C. (2003). Disorders of memory. In Office Practice of Neurology, edited by M.A. Samuels and S. Fenske. New York: Churchill Livingston.

Reiman, E.M., R.J. Caselli, L.S. Yun, K. Chen, D. Bandy, S. Minoshima, S.N. Thibodeau, and D. Osborne. (1996). Preclinical evidence of Alzheimer's disease in persons homozygous for the E4 allele for apolipoprotein E. *N Engl J Med* 334(12):752–758.

Silverman, D.H., G.W. Small, C.Y. Chang, C.S. Lu, M.A. Kung De Aburto, W. Chen, J. Czernin, S.I. Rapoport, P. Pietrini, G.E. Alexander, M.B. Schapiro, W.J. Jagust, J.M. Hoffman, K.A. Welsh-Bohmer, A. Alavi, C.M. Clark, E. Salmon, M.J. de Leon, R. Mielke, J.L. Cummings, A.P. Kowell, S.S. Gambhir, C.K. Hoh, and M.E. Phelps. (2001). Positron emission tomography in evaluation of dementia: regional brain metabolism and long-term outcome. *JAMA* 286:2120–2127.

Sliwinski, M., R.B. Lipton, H. Buschke, and W. Stewart. (1996). The effects of preclinical dementia on estimates of normal cognitive functioning in aging. *J Gerontol B Psychol Sci Soc Sci* 51(4):217–225.

Small, G.W., A. LaRue, S. Komo, A. Kaplan, and M.A. Mandelkern. (1995). Predictors of cognitive change in middle-aged and older adults with memory loss. *Am J Psychiatry* 152:1757–1764.

Smith, G., R.J. Ivnik, R.C. Petersen, J.F. Malec, E. Kokmen, and E. Tangalos. (1991). Age-associated memory impairment diagnoses: problems of reliability and concerns for terminology. *Psychol Aging* 6(4):551–558.

Weintraub, S. (2000). Neuropsychological assessment of mental state. In Principles of Behavioral and Cognitive Neurology, edited by M.-M. Mesulam (pp. 121–173). New York: Oxford Press University.

Welsh, K., N. Butters, J. Hughes, R. Mohs, and A. Heyman. (1991). Detection of abnormal memory decline in mild cases of Alzheimer's disease using CERAD neuropsychological measures. *Arch Neurol* 48(3):278–281.

Xu, Y., C.R. Jack Jr., P.C. O'Brien, E. Kokmen, G.E. Smith, R.J. Ivnik, B.F. Boeve, E.G. Tangalos, and R.C. Petersen. (2000). Usefulness of MRI measures of entorhinal cortex versus hippocampus in AD. *Neurology* 54(9):1760–1767.

CHAPTER **12**

Treatment of Mild Cognitive Impairment and Prospects for Prevention of Alzheimer's Disease

DAVID S. KNOPMAN

The therapeutic era of Alzheimer's disease (AD) began in the 1980s with a good deal of naivete about the goals of therapy and the means to achieve success. Patients with diagnosed AD were naturally the subjects for initial clinical trials. Initial expectations for discovery of short-term improvements were not realized. Gains in function were particularly difficult to document, in part because patients with diagnosed dementia are already quite constrained in what they are allowed to do. The realization that clinically meaningful benefits would be difficult to produce in mild to moderately demented individuals was somewhat disheartening. Incorporation of milder patients into clinical trials seemed necessary to uncover more convincing and clinically meaningful benefits. Moreover, interested parties demanded that benefits of anti-AD drug therapies be placed in terms more transparent than changes in cognitive test scores. It was then that clinical trialists in AD therapeutics took notice of mild cognitive impairment.

Therapeutic interventions for mild cognitive impairment (MCI) have expanded dramatically in the past few years. The U.S. Food and Drug Administration has not yet clarified whether MCI will be designated as a defined indication for therapy, but it seems likely that this will occur. Despite the uncertainty of its regulatory status, a number of agents are currently being evaluated in MCI populations. Drug therapy in MCI offers several notable advantages. Patients with MCI are much milder and higher functioning than are individuals with established dementia due to AD. As a consequence, stabilization of function in an individual with MCI has greater benefits, both for the individual and for society. As for measuring results, a therapy's ability to delay the decline to dementia is an appealing and convincing outcome that is far easier to demonstrate in an MCI population than it is in a completely asymptomatic population.

The goal of this review is to describe some of the therapeutic classes that are currently being tested in MCI patients or are being contemplated for use.

CHOLINESTERASE INHIBITOR DRUGS

Initial autopsy-based neurochemical studies in the late 1970s demonstrated deficits in the enzymes responsible for synthesis of AD (Davies and Maloney, 1976; Perry et al., 1978). Subsequent studies demonstrated the principal locations of the cholinergic projection neurons—the septum, diagonal band, and nucleus basalis—lateral and anterior to the hypothalamus exhibited marked cell loss in AD (Whitehouse et al., 1982; Saper et al., 1985; Rasool et al., 1986). Imaging of acetylcholinesterase in the human brain in situ (Kuhl et al., 1999) has provided evidence for in situ declines in cholinergic function in patients with established mild to moderate AD.

Recently, with the increasing focus on treating earlier in the disease process, clinical pathological studies have evaluated the cholinergic deficits in patients with mild AD. Davis et al. (1999) found that levels of choline acetyltransferase were not significantly lower in mild AD patients than in nondemented age-matched controls. Others have reported that numbers of nucleus basalis neurons are lower in MCI patients than in nondemented elderly (Mufson et al., 2000). The status of the cholinergic system, especially in the hippocampus, in MCI offers conflicting predictions about the chances for success of cholinergic therapies. If there is no cholinergic deficit in MCI, or if it is covered by compensatory mechanisms, therapeutic intervention may be of little value. Alternatively, if the cholinergic system was deficient but still capable of compensation, perhaps the boost provided by cholinesterase inhibitors might be more effective at that stage than at later phases of deterioration of the system. Thus, the potential for therapeutic benefits from cholinesterase inhibitors (ChEIs) in MCI patients may or may not be of the same magnitude as it has proven to be in established AD. It is useful to review the effects of ChEIs in mild to moderate AD in order to understand what might occur in MCI.

Although tacrine (Knapp et al., 1994) was the first of the cholinesterase inhibitors to be marketed, its short half-life and hepatotoxicity foiled its chances for success. This opened the door for several other agents. By the end of 2000, pivotal trials for donepezil (Rogers et al., 1998; Burns et al., 1999), rivastigmine (Corey-Bloom et al., 1998; Rosler et al., 1999), metrifonate (Cummings et al., 1998; Morris et al., 1998), and galantamine (Raskind et al., 2000; Tariot et al., 2000; Wilcock et al., 2000) had been published. The development of metrifonate was suspended after reports of muscle weakness surfaced in clinical trials, leaving donepezil, rivastigmine, and galantamine as the ChEI agents for 2001.

What is the effect of ChEI therapy on mild to moderate AD? The lines of evidence that address the effect size of the ChEIs include the data from the various 6-month clinical trials, data from open-label long-term extension studies (Rogers and Friedhoff, 1998), and a recently reported 1-year study (Mohs et al., 2001).

In the clinical trials that were approximately 6 months in duration, the differences between the placebo-treated patients and the ChEI patients have fallen in a range of 2.5 to 5 points on the Alzheimer's Disease Assessment Scale (ADAS-cog) (Rosen et al., 1984). The ADAS-cog is a widely used mental status assessment instrument that has been the standard in AD clinical trials over the years. From natural history studies and the clinical trials themselves, the drug–placebo differences correspond to about 6 to 9 months of delay of symptoms. Support for this general time frame as standing for the magnitude of the ChEI effect size comes from open-label long-term extension studies with donepezil (Rogers and Friedhoff, 1998). In these long-term extension studies, the group of patients treated with ChEI had higher test scores on the ADAS-cog on follow-up that at baseline, until approximately 35 to 40 weeks of treatment. In contrast, the placebo groups in the earlier portions of the same studies declined below their baseline assessments of the ADAS-cog in about 6 weeks. The interpretation of such data must be qualified by the fact that subjects in the open-label phase of the study were unblinded. However, at the point of transition from the double-blind phase to the open-label phase of such studies, dose reductions generally occurred.

Mohs and colleagues (2001) devised a trial design using donepezil in which 1-year placebo-controlled data were produced. In this study, they randomized subjects at baseline to either donepezil or placebo. The endpoint of the study was defined as a decline in activities of daily living of a certain amount. If subjects reached that endpoint, the primary outcome measure of the trial, they were withdrawn from the blinded study medication and offered open-label donepezil. In this clever way, an inactive treatment could be included in a 1-year study for comparison purposes but with the reassurance for participating subjects that an approved treatment would be available if they experienced decline in function. The main result of this study was to show that compared to placebo, the median time at which 50% of donepezil-treated subjects reached endpoint was 5 months later. At the 48-week point, 51% of donepezil-treated patients had not declined functionally, whereas only 38% of placebo-treated subjects had not declined functionally.

One recently published study of donepezil was conducted by investigators with no ties to the pharmaceutical manufacturer (Greenberg et al., 2000). This trial might be considered as the most robust test of the efficacy of donepezil. The study was underpowered (i.e., too few subjects to guarantee that an effect size like that previously seen would be "significant") and short in duration, and it used a low dose of donepezil. Even at donepezil at the 5 mg per day dose level, donepezil patients had higher ADAS-cog scores than did the placebo-treated patients (2.17 ± 0.98 points), which is comparable to what was seen in the course of longer studies. Of the 51 patients exposed to donepezil, 5 developed nausea, 3 diarrhea, and 3 agitation. None of these resulted in drug discontinuation.

The dosing of ChEIs has been limited by gastrointestinal side effects, but there is evidence that the maximally tolerated dosage levels might be more effective for improving brain function. Kuhl et al. (2000) showed that donepezil at 10 mg saturated only a fraction (27%) of the cerebral acetylcholinesterase, as measured by PET imaging. In contrast, acute administration of physostigmine intravenously resulted in 52% inhibition. The finding implies that currently recommended doses of donepezil may not be achieving the highest possible cortical acetylcholinesterase inhibition and that higher doses of donepezil might have greater clinical effects. Similar experiments have not been reported for rivastigmine or galantamine.

The use of cognitive test scores to judge efficacy of anti-AD drugs has been one of the cornerstones of the anti-dementia drug approval process in the United States over the past 10 years. During this time, there has been criticism and concern that additional features of AD need to be presented in outcome assessments. In particular, performance on activities of daily living has been considered by European pharmaceutical regulators to be equally relevant. The more recent traditionally designed studies, including those published in the past 2 years, have invariably included a measure of activities of daily living. Donepezil (Burns et al., 1999), rivastigmine (Rosler et al., 1999), and galantamine (Raskind et al., 2000; Tariot et al., 2000) have all demonstrated differences compared to placebo on these scales. An interesting phenomenon has been observed consistently. Whereas the cognitive scales usually have detected some improvements in test scores in the ChEI-treated subjects, the functional scales generally show lack of decline, but no improvement. In other words, caregivers, who complete the functional scales, either do not observe improvement or they do not allow their patient family member the opportunity to perform tasks that they had not been able to do before entering the trial. Probably both explanations are operative. The effects of the ChEIs are not large enough to actually improve function in a majority of subjects. However, the absence of decline can be appreciated by caregivers. As shown by the Mohs et al. (2001) study, the magnitude of the ChEI effect size on function is quite similar to the estimate derived from the cognitive tests.

Evidence has also emerged that the ChEI drugs may have effects on reducing the incidence of some of the neuropsychiatric (NP) symptoms in AD (Morris et al., 1998; Raskind et al., 1999). It is more difficult to assess the effect size of the ChEIs on this domain of function. Irritability, profound apathy, paranoia, anxiety, and the like are common emergent NP symptoms in the course of AD. Because the entry criteria for AD clinical trials do not specify a minimum level of existing symptomatology, a particular clinical trial may have many subjects with existing NP symptoms or very few. The amount of NP symptomatology that emerges over the course of the trial is likely to be related to the amount at baseline. Therefore, comparability across trials in terms of amount of behavior emerging is very difficult. Moreover, some patients never experience NP symptoms. ChEIs suppress NP symptoms, but by how much, for how long, and for which type of NP symptoms are not yet resolved. Open-label data also exist (Mega et al., 1999).

Our knowledge of the breadth of the toxicity of the ChEI drugs has been little modified by the newer studies (with the exception of the metrifonate studies). In a dose-related fashion, gastrointestinal side effects such as nausea, diarrhea, vomiting, and anorexia occur in a subset of patients. These side effects are more likely with more rapid dose escalation regimens, and less likely when the dose titration is carried out over many weeks. With the exception of metrifonate and the apparent problems with muscle weakness at high doses, no unexpected adverse events have yet appeared with the generation of ChEIs that followed tacrine. Differences between donepezil, galantamine, and rivastigmine in rates of nausea, diarrhea, and vomiting are somewhat difficult to interpret when the data are taken from clinical trials that employed different dose-escalation strategies. Rivastigmine studies generally employed weekly dose escalations and forced dose escalations to the maximally tolerated dosages. The 24-week donepezil trials, in contrast, started subjects at 5 mg per day for 4 weeks before instituting the 10 mg per day dose. Moreover, 10 mg per day of donepezil is probably not the maximally tolerated dose for the vast majority of AD patients. However, taking the adverse event profiles of the drugs at their face values, rivastigmine appears to have the highest rate of gastrointestinal side effects, while donepezil has the lowest and galantamine is intermediate.

The prospects for efficacy of ChEI drugs in MCI cannot be predicted at this time. Even though the ChEI class has proven to be of benefit in mild to moderate AD, it is not assured that they will show benefits in MCI. All three ChEIs are either part of trials using mild cognitive impairment subjects or will be. In the donepezil–vitamin E MCI trial being conducted in the Alzheimer's Disease Cooperative Study (ADCS), 720 subjects will be enrolled by November 2000 and followed for a total of 3 years. The entry criteria for the ADCS trial require the subjects to have objective memory loss, intact nonmemory cognitive functions, and independence in activities of daily living. The endpoint of the study is the development of a diagnosis of AD.

STRATEGIES AIMED AT β-AMYLOID PROCESSING

The β-amyloid (Aβ) peptide is a 40 to 42 amino acid fragment of the Alzheimer precursor protein (APP). The fate of the APP is determined by the actions of three secretases that cleave it into different fragments. In the past several years, it has become clear that the overactivity of the β or γ secretases, or of an underactivity of the α secretase could be responsible for excess Aβ production. The finding that patients with familial AD due to mutations in the presenilin genes had elevated levels of Aβ in their brains suggested that presenilin was somehow involved in the trafficking of APP (Scheuner et al., 1996; Hardy, 1997). Selkoe's laboratory (Xia et al., 1998; Wolfe et al., 1999) was among the first to provide evidence that presenilin could be the γ secretase. Subsequently, questions have been raised as to whether presenilin itself possesses the secretase activity or whether it is simply very tightly linked to the actual molecule with the enzymatic activity (Li et al., 2000). However, the story is quite compelling that presenilin is involved in the production of excess Aβ peptide. Mutations in the presenilin gene are assumed to produce a gain in function of γ secretase, thereby generating the higher loads of Aβ observed in models of presenilin mutants (Duff et al., 1996).

In late 1999, a research group at Amgen (Vassar et al., 1999) reported their success in identifying the β secretase, one of the key enzymes involved in the cleavage of the APP. Shortly thereafter, other groups (Hussain et al., 1999; Sinha et al., 1999; Yan et al., 1999) reported a replication of the finding. The β secretase is a membrane-bound aspartyl protease that is localized intracellularly in the Golgi apparatus and endosomes.

Armed with the knowledge about a prime target for preventing AD at the molecular level, initial human studies of such agents are in phase I testing as of 2002. Important questions about safety must of course be answered first. Ultimately, if these agents prove to be safe, trials meant to prove efficacy will have to be designed and executed. Whether these will involve studies in symptomatic AD patients or MCI patients remains to be seen. Trials in symptomatic AD patients will be the first to be carried out, as they involve the smallest number of subjects and are of the shortest duration. However, trials of secretase inhibitors in symptomatic AD patients run the risk of failing to show an effect in what amounts to advanced AD pathology.

IMMUNIZATION WITH AMYLOID PEPTIDE

Schenk and colleagues (1999) showed dramatic beneficial effects of monthly intraperitoneal injections of the $A\beta$ peptide itself into transgenic mice that carried the APP 717 mutation (Games et al., 1995) and that developed $A\beta$-centered neuritic plaques by 1 year of age. The APP-717 transgenic mice do not develop deficits in learning or other measurable behavioral functions, so that no "clinical" effects on the mice from the immunization were present. However, the neuropathological differences between the immunized and nonimmunized mice were quite dramatic. With immunizations near birth, $A\beta$ pathology was virtually prevented when the mice were sacrificed at 18 months of age. Schenk et al. also showed that immunizations at 11 months of age produced nearly as dramatic results. Weiner et al. (2000) reported replication of the findings, but in this latter study, $A\beta$ peptide was delivered to the mice via intranasal administration. Weiner et al. administered synthetic human $A\beta$ peptide via the nasal mucosa on a weekly basis between the ages of approximately 5 and 12 months to the Games et al. (1995) APP transgenic mouse. Treated mice had a lower plaque burden, as well as other indications of less active pathology: "decreased local microglial and astrocytic activation, decreased neuritic dystrophy" and the presence of serum anti-Aβ antibodies (Weiner et al., 2000). Subsequently, using a different mouse model, several other groups have shown that immunization prevented cognitive dysfunction in APP-transgenic mice (Chen et al., 2000; Janus et al., 2000; Morgan et al., 2000). Unfortunately, in human clinical trials, the immunization approach was associated with important toxicity.

ESTROGEN TREATMENT

Despite a sound basis in epidemiological studies and basic neuroscience, expectations for estrogen as a treatment for symptomatic AD suffered serious blows with the publication of two negative studies. The larger of the two involved over 120 women with mild AD (Mulnard et al., 2000). The study was of a year's duration. Carried out by the NIH-funded AD Cooperative Study, estrogen (in the form of orally administered equine estrogens) had no effect on cognitive function or any other measure of the disease. This study was notable for requiring participants to have previously had a hysterectomy in order to allow estrogen to be used without adding progesterone to protect the uterus and cervix against the carcinogenic actions of unopposed estrogen on these tissues. None of the outcome measures favored estrogen. On the global change rating, 80% of estrogen-treated women declined over 1 year, compared to 74% of placebo-treated women. On the ADAS-cog, estrogen-treated women actually declined slightly more than placebo-treated women: 5.6 versus 3.6 points over 12 months. A smaller study from a few centers similarly found no benefits for estrogen in AD (Henderson et al., 2000). This latter study had only 36 women who were evaluable after 16 weeks of therapy.

Prevention studies with estrogen that have recruited cognitively normal subjects are ongoing. In one that is still early in its enrollment phase, women without cognitive impairment but with family histories of AD are being recruited for a prevention trial (Sano, personal communication). In the other, the Women's Health Initiative Memory study (Shumaker and Rapp, 1996), 8000 women treated with estrogen plus progesterone or placebo are being followed for many years to establish definitively whether estrogen plus progesterone has any protective effects against the development of AD. As of 2002, active treatment ended in this trial, but the subjects will continue to be followed. Because of the negative results for symptomatic AD and the ongoing prevention studies, it seems unlikely that any studies of estrogen with MCI subjects will be carried out in the foreseeable future.

ANTI-INFLAMMATORY DRUGS

There has been substantial interest in anti-inflammatory drugs as treatment for AD. A series of epidemiological studies have shown that nonsteroidal anti-inflammatory drugs (NSAID) use was associated with a lower incidence of AD. Unfortunately, the clinical trial data have failed to support the hypothesis. A 1-year trial of low-dose prednisone (1 month of 20 mg per day followed by 11 months of 10 mg per day) versus placebo in 138 symptomatic mild to moderate AD patients did not support the idea that an anti-inflammatory drug affected the symptoms of AD (Aisen et al., 2000). Conducted by the ADCS, this study failed to show any beneficial effects for this agent on cognitive test scores (ADAS-cog), global ratings (CDR sum of boxes), or behavioral ratings. One of the criticisms of the study was that the dose of prednisone was too low to have an inhibitory effect on the inflammatory processes that are believed to be occurring in the AD brain. However, it was believed to be the highest dose for which safety over a 1-year period could be assured.

A small study with the nonsteroidal anti-inflammatory drug diclofenac failed to demonstrate any differences between placebo-treated and diclofenac-treated patients except in drop-out rates (Scharf et al., 1999). Half of the NSAID-treated subjects withdrew before the end of the 25-week trial.

A multinational 1-year trial of celecoxib in AD unfortunately proved to be negative (Sainati et al., 2000). Results were presented only in abstract form, but the clear result was that there was no difference between placebo-treated and celecoxib-treated patients in the intent-to-treat population after 52 weeks of therapy.

Three trials are currently ongoing that involve NSAID drugs. One is occurring in a symptomatic AD population and is comparing naproxen and the cyclo-oxygenase II inhibitor, rofecoxib. Another rofecoxib study is being carried out in an MCI population. A third study using naproxen and rofecoxib is being tested in normal individuals for its ability to prevent AD.

OTHER STRATEGIES

Several studies have suggested that lipid-lowering strategies might be of value in the treatment of AD. A recent meta-analysis (Wolozin et al., 2000) suggested that treatment with cholesterol-lowering agents was associated with a reduced risk for AD. In an incidence study from the Netherlands (Kalmijn et al., 1997), dietary total fat intake (RR = 2.4) was associated with incident dementia. In contrast, serum LDL cholesterol levels were not associated with risk for AD but, rather, only for dementia with stroke (Moroney et al., 1999). Currently, clinical trials with cholesterol-lowering agents as treatments for symptomatic AD are either being planned or are actually enrolling subjects.

Hypertension is a risk factor for cognitive decline and dementia (Launer et al., 1995; Glynn et al., 1999). A trial of anti-hypertensives in Europe showed that treatment with nitrendipine (calcium-channel blocker) resulted in a reduced incidence of dementia (Forette et al., 1998). A similar trial in the United Kingdom, however, failed to show a benefit in terms of change in cognitive function over time (Prince et al., 1996).

CONCLUSIONS

MCI may be the strategy that helps the field of AD therapeutics bridge the gap between treatments that might be efficacious in symptomatic patients and those who are cognitively normal. It is conceivable that clinical trials in MCI subjects might prove more informative than trials in symptomatic AD patients because of the earlier stage of pathology represented by MCI. Several trials involving MCI subjects are underway (Table 12–1).

Disclosure

Dr. Knopman has served as an ad hoc paid consultant in the past two years to Eisai/Pfizer, Cortex, and Bristol-Myers-Squibb. Dr. Knopman and his family do not own stock or have equity interests in any pharmaceutical or biotechnology company whose agents were mentioned in this article.

Table 12–1. Agents Being Tested in Subjects with Mild Cognitive Impairment

Agent	Mechanism of action	Duration	Outcome measure
Vitamin E	Antioxidant	3 years	Alzheimer's Disease
Donepezil	Cholinesterase inhibitor	3 years	Alzheimer's Disease
Rivastigmine	Cholinesterase inhibitor	2–3 years	Alzheimer's Disease
Galantamine	Cholinesterase inhibitor	2–3 years	Alzheimer's Disease
Rofecoxib		2–3 years	Dementia
Donepezil	Cholinesterase inhibitor	6 months	Change in cognitive function
Piracetam	Cholinergic agonist	1 year	Change in cognitive function
CX-516	AMPA* receptor modulator	4 weeks	Change in cognitive function

*a-amino-3-hydroxy-5-methyl-4isoxazol propionic acid.

References

Aisen, P.S., K.L. Davis, J.D. Berg, K. Schafer, K. Campbell, R.G. Thomas, M.F. Weiner, M.R. Farlow, M. Sano, M. Grundman, and L.J. Thal. (2000). A randomized controlled trial of prednisone in Alzheimer's disease. Alzheimer's Disease Cooperative Study. *Neurology* 54:588–593.

Burns, A., M. Rossor, J. Hecker, S. Gauthier, H. Petit, H. Miller, S.L. Rogers, and L.T. Friedhoff. (1999). The effects of Donepezil in Alzheimer's disease: results from a multinational trial. *Dement Geriatr Cogn Disord* 10: 237–244.

Chen, G., K.S. Chen, J. Knox, J. Inglis, A. Bernard, S.J. Martin, A. Justice, L. McConlogue, D. Games, S.B. Freedman, and R.G. Morris. (2000). A learning deficit related to age and β-amyloid plaques in a mouse model of Alzheimer's disease. *Nature* 408:975–979.

Corey-Bloom, J., R. Anand, J. Veach, and the ENA 713 B352 Study Group. (1998). A randomized trial evaluating the efficacy and safety of ENA 713 (rivastigmine tartrate), a new acetylcholinesterase inhibitor, in patients with mild to moderately severe Alzheimer's disease. *Int J Geriatric Psychopharmacol* 1:55–65.

Cummings, J.L., P.A. Cyrus, F. Bieber, J. Mas, J. Orazem, and B. Gulanski. (1998). Metrifonate treatment of the cognitive deficits of Alzheimer's disease. *Neurology* 50:1214–1221.

Davies, P., and A.J. Maloney. (1976). Selective loss of central cholinergic neurons in Alzheimer's disease. *Lancet* 2:1403.

Davis, K.L., R.C. Mohs, D. Marin, D.P. Purohit, D.P. Perl, M. Lantz, G. Austin, and V. Haroutunian. (1999). Cholinergic markers in elderly patients with early signs of Alzheimer disease. *JAMA* 281:1401–1406.

Duff, K., C. Eckman, C. Zehr, X. Yu, C.M. Prada, J. Perez-tur, M. Hutton, L. Buee, Y. Harigaya, D. Yager, D. Morgan, M.N. Gordon, L. Holcomb, L. Refolo, B. Zenk, J. Hardy, and S. Younkin. (1996). Increased amyloid-β42(43) in brains of mice expressing mutant presenilin 1. *Nature* 383:710–713.

Forette, F., M.L. Seux, J.A. Staessen, L. Thijs, W.H. Birkenhager, M.R. Babarskiene, S. Babeanu, A. Bossini, B. Gil-Extremera, X. Girerd, T. Laks, E. Lilov, V. Moisseyev, J. Tuomilehto, H. Vanhanen, J. Webster, Y. Yodfat, and R. Fagard. (1998). Prevention of dementia in randomised double blind placebo-controlled systolic hypertension in Europe (Syst-Eur) trial. *Lancet* 352:1347–1351.

Games, D., D. Adams, R. Alessandrini, R. Barbour, P. Berthelette, C. Blackwell, T. Carr, J. Clemens, T. Donaldson, F. Gillespie, et al. (1995). Alzheimer-type neuropathology in transgenic mice overexpressing V717F β-amyloid precursor protein. *Nature* 373:523–527.

Glynn, R.J., L.A. Beckett, L.E. Hebert, M.C. Morris, P.A. Scherr, and D.A. Evans. (1999). Current and remote blood pressure and cognitive decline. *JAMA* 281:438–445.

Greenberg, S.M., M.K. Tennis, L.B. Brown, T. Gomez-Isla, D.L. Hayden, D.A. Schoenfeld, K.L. Walsh, C. Corwin, K.R. Daffner, P. Friedman, M.E. Meadows, R.A. Sperling, and J.H. Growdon. (2000). Donepezil therapy in clinical practice: a randomized crossover study. *Arch Neurol* 57:94–99.

Hardy, J. (1997). Amyloid, the presenilins and Alzheimer's disease. *Trends Neurosci* 20:154–159.

Henderson, V.W., A. Paganini-Hill, B.L. Miller, R.J. Elble, P.F. Reyes, D. Shoupe, C.A. McCleary, R.A. Klein, A.M. Hake, and M.R. Farlow. (2000). Estrogen for Alzheimer's disease in women: randomized, double-blind, placebo-controlled trial. *Neurology* 54:295–301.

Hussain, I., D. Powell, D.R. Howlett, D.G. Tew, T.D. Meek, C. Chapman, I.S. Gloger, K.E. Murphy, C.D. Southan, D.M. Ryan, T.S. Smith, D.L. Simmons, F.S. Walsh, C. Dingwall, and G. Christie. (1999). Identification of a novel aspartic protease (Asp 2) as β-secretase. *Mol Cell Neurosci* 14:419–427.

Janus, C., J. Pearson, J. McLaurin, P.M. Mathews, Y. Jiang, S.D. Schmidt, M.A. Chishti, P. Horne, D. Heslin, J. French, H.T. Mount, R.A. Nixon, M. Mercken, C. Bergeron, P.E. Fraser, P. St. George-Hyslop, and D. Westaway. (2000). A β peptide immunization reduces behavioural impairment and plaques in a model of Alzheimer's disease. *Nature* 408: 979–982.

Kalmijn, S., L.J. Launer, A. Ott, J.C. Witteman, A. Hofman, and M.M. Breteler. (1997). Dietary fat intake and the risk of incident dementia in the Rotterdam study. *Ann Neurol* 42:776–782.

Knapp, M.J., D.S. Knopman, P.R. Solomon, W.W. Pendlebury, C.S. Davis, and S.I. Gracon. (1994). A 30-week randomized controlled trial of high-dose tacrine in patients with Alzheimer's disease. *JAMA* 271:985–991.

Kuhl, D.E., R.A. Koeppe, S. Minoshima, S.E. Snyder, E.P. Ficaro, N.L. Foster, K.A. Frey, and M.R. Kilbourn. (1999). In vivo mapping of cerebral acetylcholinesterase activity in aging and Alzheimer's disease. *Neurology* 52: 691–699.

Kuhl, D.E., S. Minoshima, K.A. Frey, N.L. Foster, M.R. Kilbourn, and R.A. Koeppe. (2000). Limited donepezil inhibition of acetylcholinesterase measured with positron emission tomography in living Alzheimer cerebral cortex. *Ann Neurol* 48:391–395.

Launer, L.J., K. Masaki, H. Petrovitch, D. Foley, and R.J. Havlik. (1995). The association between midlife blood pressure levels and late-life cognitive function. *JAMA* 274:1846–1851.

Li, Y.M., M.T. Lai, M. Xu, Q. Huang, J. DiMuzio-Mower, M.K. Sardana, X.P. Shi, K.C. Yin, J.A. Shafer, and S.J. Gardell. (2000). Presenilin 1 is linked with γ-secretase activity in the detergent solubilized state. *Proc Natl Acad Sci USA* 97:6138–6143.

Mega, M.S., D.M. Masterman, S.M. O'Connor, T.R. Barclay, and J.L. Cummings. (1999). The spectrum of behavioral responses to cholinesterase inhibitor therapy in Alzheimer disease. *Arch Neurol* 56:1388–1393.

Mohs, R.C., R.S. Doody, J.C. Morris, J.R. Ieni, S.L. Rogers, C.A. Perdomo, R.D. Pratt, and the "312" Study Group. (2001). A 1-year placebo-controlled preservation of function survival study of donepezil in AD patients. *Neurology* 57:481–488.

Morgan, D., D.M. Diamond, P.E. Gottschall, K.E. Ugen, C. Dickey, J. Hardy, K. Duff, P. Jantzen, G. DiCarlo, D. Wilcock, K. Connor, J. Hatcher, C. Hope, M. Gordon, and G.W. Arendash. (2000). A β peptide vaccination prevents memory loss in an animal model of Alzheimer's disease. *Nature* 408:982–985.

Moroney, J.T., M.X. Tang, L. Berglund, S. Small, C. Merchant, K. Bell, Y. Stern, and R. Mayeux. (1999). Low-density lipoprotein cholesterol and the risk of dementia with stroke. *JAMA* 282:254–260.

Morris, J.C., P.A. Cyrus, J. Orazem, J. Mas, F. Bieber, B.B. Ruzicka, and B. Gulanski. (1998). Metrifonate benefits cognitive, behavioral, and global function in patients with Alzheimer's disease. *Neurology* 50:1222–1230.

Mufson, E.J., S.Y. Ma, E.J. Cochran, D.A. Bennett, L.A. Beckett, S. Jaffar, H.U. Saragovi, and J.H. Kordower. (2000). Loss of nucleus basalis neurons containing trkA immunoreactivity in individuals with mild cognitive impairment and early Alzheimer's disease. *J Comp Neurol* 427:19–30.

Mulnard, R.A., C.W. Cotman, C. Kawas, C.H. van Dyck, M. Sano, R. Doody, E. Koss, E. Pfeiffer, S. Jin, A. Gamst, M. Grundman, R. Thomas, and L.J. Thal. (2000). Estrogen replacement therapy for treatment of mild to moderate Alzheimer disease: a randomized controlled trial. *JAMA* 283:1007–1015.

Perry, E.K., B.E. Tomlinson, G. Blessed, K. Bergmann, P.H. Gibson, and R.H. Perry. (1978). Correlation of cholinergic abnormalities with senile plaques and mental test scores in senile dementia. *Br Med J* 2:1457–1459.

Prince, M.J., A.S. Bird, R.A. Blizard, and A.H. Mann. (1996). Is the cognitive function of older patients affected by antihypertensive treatment? Results from 54 months of the Medical Research Council's trial of hypertension in older adults. *Br Med J* 312:801–805.

Raskind, M.A., P.A. Cyrus, B.B. Ruzicka, and B.I. Gulanski. (1999). The effects of metrifonate on the cognitive, behavioral, and functional performance of Alzheimer's disease patients. *J Clin Psychiatry* 60:318–325.

Raskind, M.A., E.R. Peskind, T. Wessel, and W. Yuan. (2000). Galantamine in AD: a 6-month randomized, placebo-controlled trial with a 6-month extension. *Neurology* 54:2261–2268.

Rasool, C.G., C.N. Svendsen, and D.J. Selkoe. (1986). Neurofibrillary degeneration of cholinergic and noncholinergic neurons of the basal forebrain in Alzheimer's disease. *Ann Neurol* 20:482–488.

Rogers, S.L., and L.T. Friedhoff. (1998). Long-term efficacy and safety of donepezil in the treatment of Alzheimer's disease: an interim analysis of the results of a U.S. multicentre open label extension study. *Eur Neuropsychopharmacol* 8:67–75.

Rogers, S.L., M.R. Farlow, R.S. Doody, R. Mohs, and L.T. Friedhoff. (1998). A 24-week, double-blind, placebo-controlled trial of donepezil in patients with Alzheimer's disease. *Neurology* 50:136–145.

Rosen, W.G., R.C. Mohs, and K.L. Davis. (1984). A new rating scale for Alzheimer's disease. *Am J Psychiatry* 141:1356–1364.

Rosler, M., R. Anand, A. Cicin-Sain, S. Gauthier, Y. Agid, P. Dal-Bianco, H.B. Stahelin, R. Hartman, and M. Gharabawi. (1999). Efficacy and safety of rivastigmine in patients with Alzheimer's disease: international randomised controlled trial. *Br Med J* 318:633–640.

Sainati, S.M., D.M. Ingram, S. Talwalker, and G.S. Geis. (2000). Results of a double-blind, randomized, placebo-controlled study of celecoxib in the treatment of progression of Alzheimer's disease. *Sixth International Stockholm/Springfield Symposium on Advances in Alzheimer Therapy April 5–8*, 2000:180.

Saper, C.B., D.C. German, and C.L. White. (1985). Neuronal pathology in the nucleus basalis and associated cell groups in senile dementia of the Alzheimer's type: possible role in cell loss. *Neurology* 35:1089–1095.

Scharf, S., A. Mander, A. Ugoni, F. Vajda, and N. Christophidis. (1999). A double-blind, placebo-controlled trial of diclofenac/misoprostol in Alzheimer's disease. *Neurology* 53:197–201.

Schenk, D., R. Barbour, W. Dunn, G. Gordon, H. Grajeda, T. Guido, K. Hu, J. Huang, K. Johnson-Wood, K. Khan, D. Kholodenko, M. Lee, Z. Liao, I. Lieberburg, R. Motter, L. Mutter, F. Soriano, G. Shopp, N. Vasquez, C. Vandevert, S. Walker, M. Wogulis, T. Yednock, D. Games, and P. Seubert. (1999). Immunization with amyloid-β attenuates Alzheimer-disease-like pathology in the PDAPP mouse. *Nature* 400:173–177.

Scheuner, D., C. Eckman, M. Jensen, X. Song, M. Citron, N. Suzuki, T.D. Bird, J. Hardy, M. Hutton, W. Kukull, E. Larson, E. Levy-Lahad, M. Viitanen, E. Peskind, P. Poorkaj, G. Schellenberg, R. Tanzi, W. Wasco, L. Lannfelt, D. Selkoe, and S. Younkin. (1996). Secreted amyloid β-protein similar to that in the senile plaques of Alzheimer's disease is increased in vivo by the presenilin 1 and 2 and APP mutations linked to familial Alzheimer's disease. *Nat Med* 2:864–870.

Shumaker, S., and S. Rapp. (1996). Hormone therapy in dementia prevention: the Womens Health Initiative memory study. *Neurobiol Aging* 17: S9.

Sinha, S., J.P. Anderson, R. Barbour, G.S. Basi, R. Caccavello, D. Davis, M. Doan, H.F. Dovey, N. Frigon, J. Hong, K. Jacobson-Croak, N. Jewett, P. Keim, J. Knops, I. Lieberburg, M. Power, H. Tan, G. Tatsuno, J. Tung, D. Schenk, P. Seubert, S.M. Suomensaari, S. Wang, D. Walker, V. John, et al. (1999). Purification and cloning of amyloid precursor protein β-secretase from human brain. *Nature* 402:537–540.

Tariot, P.N., P.R. Solomon, J.C. Morris, P. Kershaw, S. Lilienfeld, and C. Ding. (2000). A 5-month, randomized, placebo-controlled trial of galantamine in AD. *Neurology* 54:2269–2276.

Vassar, R., B.D. Bennett, S. Babu-Khan, S. Kahn, E.A. Mendiaz, P. Denis, D.B. Teplow, S. Ross, P. Amarante, R. Loeloff, Y. Luo, S. Fisher, J. Fuller, S. Edenson, J. Lile, M.A. Jarosinski, A.L. Biere, E. Curran, T. Burgess, J.C. Louis, F. Collins, J. Treanor, G. Rogers, and M. Citron. (1999). β-secretase cleavage of Alzheimer's amyloid precursor protein by the transmembrane aspartic protease BACE. *Science* 286:735–741.

Weiner, H.L., C.A. Lemere, R. Maron, E.T. Spooner, T.J. Grenfell, C. Mori, S. Issazadeh, W.W. Hancock, and D.J. Selkoe. (2000). Nasal administration of amyloid-β peptide decreases cerebral amyloid burden in a mouse model of Alzheimer's disease. *Ann Neurol* 48:567–579.

Whitehouse, P.J., D.L. Price, R.G. Struble, A.W. Clark, J.T. Coyle, and M.R. Delon. (1982). Alzheimer's disease and senile dementia: loss of neurons in the basal forebrain. *Science* 215:1237–1239.

Wilcock, G.K., S. Lilienfeld, and E. Gaens. (2000). Efficacy and safety of galantamine in patients with mild to moderate Alzheimer's disease: multicentre randomised controlled trial. *Br Med J* 321:1445–1449.

Wolfe, M.S., W. Xia, B.L. Ostaszewski, T.S. Diehl, W.T. Kimberly, and D.J. Selkoe. (1999). Two transmembrane aspartates in presenilin-1 required for presenilin endoproteolysis and γ-secretase activity. *Nature* 398:513–517.

Wolozin, B., W. Kellman, P. Ruosseau, G.G. Celesia, and G. Siegel. (2000). Decreased prevalence of Alzheimer disease associated with 3-hydroxy-3-methyglutaryl coenzyme A reductase inhibitors. *Arch Neurol* 57:1439–1443.

Xia, W., J. Zhang, B.L. Ostaszewski, W.T. Kimberly, P. Seubert, E.H. Koo, J. Shen, and D.J. Selkoe. (1998). Presenilin 1 regulates the processing of β-amyloid precursor protein C-terminal fragments and the generation of amyloid β-protein in endoplasmic reticulum and Golgi. *Biochemistry* 37:16465–16471.

Yan, R., M.J. Bienkowski, M.E. Shuck, H. Miao, M.C. Tory, A.M. Pauley, J.R. Brashier, N.C. Stratman, W.R. Mathews, A.E. Buhl, D.B. Carter, A.G. Tomasselli, L.A. Parodi, R.L. Heinrikson, and M.E. Gurney. (1999). Membrane-anchored aspartyl protease with Alzheimer's disease β-secretase activity. *Nature* 402:533–537.

INDEX

Page numbers followed by *f* and *t* indicate figures and tables, respectively.